Guide to Paediatric Haematology Morphology

This illustrated guide to identifying or confirming blood disorders in paediatric patients presents examples of the abnormal morphology involved. Clinicians in both Haematology and Paediatrics will find this an invaluable resource.

Gillian Rozenberg, Consultant in blood film morphology, FAIMS (Life Member), FFSc (RCPA) is the Principal Medical Scientist working in the field of Diagnostic Haematology at the Prince of Wales Hospital, Sydney, Australia.

T0303918

Guide to Paediatric Haematology Morphology

Gillian Rozenberg

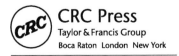

CRC Press
Taylor & Francis Group
Boca Raton London New York

CRC Press is an imprint of the
Taylor & Francis Group, an **informa** business

Designed cover image: Author

First edition published 2025
by CRC Press
2385 NW Executive Center Drive, Suite 320, Boca Raton FL 33431

and by CRC Press
4 Park Square, Milton Park, Abingdon, Oxon, OX14 4RN
CRC Press is an imprint of Taylor & Francis Group, LLC

© 2025 Gillian Rozenberg

ISBN: 9781032755373 (hbk)
ISBN: 9781032753904 (pbk)
ISBN: 9781003474432 (ebk)

DOI: 10.1201/9781003474432

Typeset in Casion
by Deanta Global Publishing Services, Chennai, India

Contents

Acknowledgements

There are a number of colleagues who I would like to thank for their assistance with the production of this book.

I would like to thank Professor Robert Lindeman, Haematologist and now currently Director of Clinical Operations for NSW Health Pathology, for allowing me access to the blood films and bone marrow films in the Haematology Laboratory and supporting me in my desire to produce this book.

My special thanks go to Martyn Palmer, a digital image artist who reviewed all 161 figures, ensuring optimum quality of all the images in this book.

Also, my thanks go to Robert Peden, a Senior Editor from Taylor & Francis Group, for his advice whilst compiling this work.

Examination of the blood film

A well-stained blood film is the key to a clear, accurate interpretation of the findings under the microscope.

Preparation of the blood film

Blood is collected into the anticoagulant ethylenediamine tetra-acetic acid (EDTA) dipotassium salt concentration of 1.5 + 0.25 mg per mL.

The ratio of blood to EDTA is critical as excess EDTA results in shrinkage and degeneration of the cells, especially the red cells.

The quality of the blood film is directly related to the materials used to produce the blood film.

The glass slide must be of a high quality. It must be pre-cleaned with a frosted end and preferably, from a safety aspect, have bevelled edges. The spreader used to produce the blood film must also be of a high quality and also have bevelled edges.

Dry the blood film immediately in front of a cold-air fan and fix in AR grade methanol. The methanol MUST be at room temperature (15–20°C), stain with a Romanowsky stain, preferably Wright's stain and cover with a glass coverslip.

Examination of the blood film

The blood film is examined systematically.

On low power (×10 objective):

- Check the tail for platelet clumping.
- Check the number and distribution of the white cells.
- Check for the presence of rouleaux and correlate with the ESR result.

On high power (×40 objective):

- Perform a white cell differential.
- Estimate and correlate the platelet count with the count issued by the blood cell analyser.
- Examine the red cells as to their size, shape and colour.

On oil immersion (×100 objective):

- Examine for the presence of malarial parasites on the thick film.
- Examine for red cell inclusions when indicated.

DOI: 10.1201/9781003474432-1

Artefactual changes seen on the blood film

Incorrect ratio of blood to EDTA.

- Excess EDTA leads to the shrinkage of the red cells.
- Moisture in the methanol produces rings in the red cells giving a false impression of hypochromasia. Ensure the methanol is stored at room temperature at ALL times.

Red cell artefact

Slow drying of the blood film.

Moisture from the atmosphere will be absorbed onto the surface of the red cells, increasing the surface area unevenly, inducing the appearance of 'pseudo' target cells.

Action of heat on the red cells:

Heat will give rise to spherocytes as well as red cell fragmentation which in turn leads to a false high platelet count.

White cell artefact

Old blood:

When blood is stored in EDTA for more than 24 hours, vacuoles will be seen in the cytoplasm of the neutrophils and monocytes. Also, the nuclei of the neutrophils become degenerate. The neutrophil lobes separate and become pyknotic. A process known as 'apoptosis.'

Poor staining

- Stain precipitate on the blood film
- Incorrect staining times
- Ratio of stain to buffer incorrect
- pH of buffer too high or too low

Crush artefact

White cells may be crushed while spreading the blood film, especially lymphocytes of lymphoproliferative disorders (CLL/SLL). Such crushed cells are known as smudge cells. This artefact may be minimised by the addition of albumin (1 drop of 30% albumin to 9 drops of blood).

Platelet artefact

- Difficult collection.

- Platelet aggregation resulting from poor venepuncture technique.
- Carefully examine the blood film, especially the tail of the film, when platelets are unexpectedly reduced.
- Platelet satellitism: Usually due to immunoglobulins potentiated by EDTA causing platelets to adhere to the neutrophils.

Red cell classification

- Both normal and pathological red cells may be distorted during spreading.
- Red cells should be examined in an area where they are just touching.
- Keep away from the tail as well as the thicker part of the film, especially if rouleaux is present.

Red cells are classified under the following:

Anisocytosis–size
- Larger cells (macrocytes) and smaller cells (microcytes).
- The red cell distribution width (RDW) is the index of anisocytosis.

Poikilocytosis–shape
- Poikilocytes are produced as a result of abnormal erythropoiesis, pathological conditions and inherited disorders.

Red cell colour
- Normochromasia
- Hypochromasia
- Hyperchromia
- Polychromasia

Significance of the red cell distribution width (RDW)

The RDW is an index of anisocytosis or variation in red cell size. It is a significant parameter in many red cell disorders and may be used as a guide in the differential diagnosis of certain anaemias.

- RDW-CV (NR < 14.5%) RDW-SD (NR < 48 fL)
- RDW increased ↑ in Fe deficiency/RDW decreased ↓ in children aged between six months and five years
- RDW ↓ in thalassaemia trait and ↑ in thalassaemia intermedia and thalassaemia major
- RDW ↑ in myelodysplastic syndrome (MDS)

Anisocytosis is reported as a degree in the variation of red cell size.
It will be either mild (+), moderate (++) or marked (+++); never report as occasional.

The presence of reticulocytes which are larger than mature red cells should be excluded when reporting the degree of anisocytosis.

A moderate degree of anisocytosis should be qualified by the presence of microcytes as well as macrocytes.

The morphological abnormalities seen in red cells on a well-spread, well-stained blood film, offer a key to the interpretation of a particular pathological condition. Conversely, certain pathological conditions may be attributed to the presence of certain red cell shapes on the blood film.

With this in mind, the morphologist must be ever mindful of the standard nomenclature used to describe these red cell shapes. The ability to recognise true red cell shapes as to those produced artificially 'in vitro' is vital to an accurate film report.

The degree used to describe red cell shapes may also have a clinical significance.

In general, the morphologist should not comment on red cell shapes occurring 'occasionally' on the blood film. A mild, moderate or marked number of red cell shapes is suggestive of a pathological condition.

The use of the term occasional may confuse the diagnosis.

Never use the term 'poikilocyte' to describe variation in red cell shape. Every red cell that is not a biconcave disc or discocyte is a poikilocyte.

QUESTION*: What am I conveying to the clinician by reporting moderate or marked poikilocytes? If there are moderate or marked red cell changes on the blood film, then report these individual changes. By reporting this way, the diagnosis will be clear to both the morphologist and the clinician.

Note to reader

Comments in *italic type* indicate areas where there is often a lack of comprehension by scientists when reporting on blood films. These comments act as a reminder for the reporting morphologist.

SECTION 1
RED CELLS

Erythrocytes in the neonate and childhood

Are they macrocytic, normocytic or microcytic (why the change in size?)

Red cell changes occurring during the first six years of life relate to physiological events which take place in the haemopoietic system. These events directly relate to the age of the child.

Erythropoiesis can be divided into three major stages. Stage 1, the first three months of life, when the red cells are macrocytic and normochromic. Stage 2, from three to six months of age, when the red cells become normocytic and normochromic and stage 3, from six months to six years of age, or sometimes even longer, when the red cells become microcytic and hypochromic.

Why are these changes occurring in red cells? How important is it to recognise these changes as being physiological and thus negating the need to perform haematological diagnostic blood tests? During the third trimester of pregnancy, red cell production in the fetus proceeds at a rate of 3–5 times that of an adult. This accelerated rate of red cell production results in fewer red cell divisions during maturation, hence the red cells of cord blood are macrocytic with a mean cell volume (MCV) ranging from 101 to 117 fL. The number of reticulocytes present in cord blood is also increased. The reticulocyte count for a full-term infant ranges from 3 to 7%. The MCV and reticulocyte count start to decline during the later period of gestation. Hence the more premature the infant the higher will be the MCV and the reticulocyte count.

Changes in the rate of erythropoiesis occur in the first few days after birth. These changes are triggered by increased delivery of oxygen to the lungs. This causes a decrease in erythropoietin (EPO) production leading to a reduction in the rate of erythropoiesis. The red cell count and the haemoglobin (Hb) fall, together with the MCV and reticulocyte count. The reticulocyte count reaches a level of 0–1% by the end of the first week. Thus, the period from three to six months of age (stage 2) is characterised by red cells that are normocytic and normochromic.

The changes in erythropoiesis which occur in the first few days after birth impact on the iron stores of the infant. During gestation there is a rapid accumulation of iron by the fetus. This accumulation occurs despite the iron status of the mother. Iron deficiency in the mother has little effect on the haemoglobin or the serum ferritin level of the newborn infant. The reduction in the rate of erythropoiesis which occurs as the result of oxygenation of the lungs is accompanied by a fall in the Hb, MCV and the reticulocyte count. Reduced erythropoiesis continues for about 6–8 weeks.

DOI: 10.1201/9781003474432-2

5

During this period, iron released from the red cell breakdown is stored in the reticu-loendothelial system and provides adequate iron stores for the first six months of life of the infant. After this period, absorption of iron becomes necessary to maintain a normal iron balance. Thus from six months to six years of age (stage 3), the red cells are characteristically microcytic and hypochromic. The ferritin level is low and will remain so until replenished by iron from an adequate diet. Often during this period, diet is unbalanced and, together with the rapid increase in body weight, replenishment of iron stores is variable. Thus, the microcytic hypochromic blood picture is dependent on the dietary intake of iron.

When iron stores have been fully replenished, erythropoiesis proceeds normally and the red cells are normocytic and normochromic. It continues so throughout healthy adult life.

Normal red cell ranges have been determined for the various age groups of child-hood. The morphologist must always refer to these ranges when deciding the need for further investigations. A low MCV may indicate iron deficiency anaemia, thal-assaemia or an abnormal haemoglobin. Consider the clinical history and the age of the patient. Also consider looking at the RDW in such a case before suggesting iron studies and haemoglobin electrophoresis. Also consider careful observation of the chemistry results; put it all together before you make a diagnosis.

Feto-maternal haemorrhage

Feto-maternal haemorrhage occurs when there is a loss of fetal red cells into the maternal circulation. It occurs in normal pregnancies or when there are obstetric- or trauma-related complications to pregnancy.

Two methods can be performed to confirm a feto-maternal haemorrhage, namely, a manual method known as the Kleihauer–Betke test and an automated method by flow cytometry using anti-fetal haemoglobin antibodies (anti-HbF).

The manual method involves making a blood film from the mother's blood and exposing it to an acid bath. The acid removes the adult haemoglobin from the adult cells but not the fetal haemoglobin from the fetal cells. The blood film is stained with eosin (a red coloured stain). When the slide is viewed under the microscope, the fetal cells appear pink while the adult cells are colourless and appear as ghost cells.

Two thousand cells are counted under the microscope and a percentage of fetal to maternal cells is calculated. This calculation ascertains the number of fetal cells in the mother's circulation.

The art of blood film morphology

Red cell reference ranges in infancy and childhood

Red cell reference ranges

Age	Hb (g/L)		RCC (x 10¹²/L)		Hct (L/L)		MCV (fL)		MCH (pg)		MCHC(g/L)		RDW-SD (fL)		RDW-CV (%)	
0-1 d	121	191	3.34	5.40	0.37	0.60	101	117	33.0	38.0	302	341	61.9	81.4	15.5	19.2
1-7 d	125	195	3.90	5.60	0.38	0.60	97	107	32.0	34.8	328	325	55.0	81.4	14.0	19.2
1-2 w	120	185	3.80	5.50	0.36	0.55	95	100	31.5	33.6	333	336	50.0	70.0	12.0	18.0
2w - 3m	102	130	3.38	3.94	0.30	0.38	84	98	29.0	33.8	333	355	39.9	56.6	12.6	16.0
3-6 m	100	122	3.39	4.86	0.28	0.36	68	85	22.6	29.7	331	351	34.0	42.4	12.0	14.8
6m – 2y	104	132	3.88	5.13	0.30	0.38	70	83	23.1	29.4	323	354	34.8	44.6	12.3	17.0
2-4 y	107	136	3.86	5.01	0.31	0.38	73	85	24.8	29.9	329	359	34.3	44.1	12.1	15.6
4-8 y	110	139	3.96	4.92	0.32	0.39	74	86	25.5	30.6	332	360	34.6	42.7	11.9	14.9
8-12 y	113	143	3.98	5.15	0.33	0.41	75	86	25.7	30.6	335	361	35.3	41.0	12.0	14.1

This chart demonstrates the reference ranges for cord blood (0–1 day) to 12 years of age. Red cell reference ranges continue until puberty (12 years of age) after which time adult red cell ranges should be quoted. The mean cell volume and the mean cell haemoglobin are an indication as to whether the red cells are normal for age.

This chart demonstrates the reference ranges for cord blood (0–1 day) to 12 years of age (puberty) when adult reference ranges are issued.

Red cell reference ranges

Age	MCV (fL)		MCH (pg)	
0-1 d	101	117	33.0	38.0
1-7 d	97	107	32.0	34.8
1-2 w	95	100	31.5	33.6
2w - 3m	84	98	29.0	33.8
3-6 m	68	85	22.6	29.7
6m – 2y	70	83	23.1	29.4
2-4 y	73	85	24.8	29.9
4-8 y	74	86	25.5	30.6
8-12 y	75	86	25.7	30.6

This is a simplified chart emphasising the changes in mean cell volume and mean cell haemoglobin ranging from 0 days to 12 years of age. Note the red cells are macrocytic at birth and gradually reduce in size towards puberty. At 12 years of age, red cell reference ranges change to adult ranges.

This is a simplified chart emphasising changes in the MCV and the mean cell haemoglobin (MCH) from 0 days to 12 years of age.

Reticulocyte reference ranges

RETICULO-CYTES %	CORD BLOOD	DAY 1	DAY 3	DAY 7	DAY 14
	3 - 7	3 - 7	1 - 3	0 - 1	0 - 1

This chart demonstrates reticulocyte counts during the first two weeks of life. Note the reticulocyte count is increased in cord blood (ranging from 3 to 7%) and gradually reduces in number until the first week in life when the count ranges from 0 to 1%.

This chart demonstrates reticulocyte counts in the first week of life.

Electron microscopic image of normal red cells

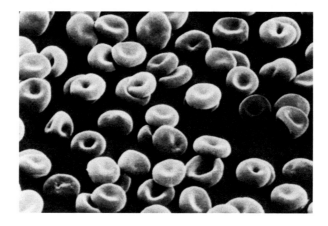

This is an electron microscopic image of normal red cells demonstrating that mature red cells are biconcave discs (×1000).

Cord blood

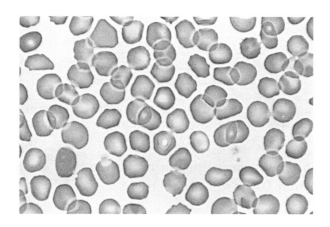

Cord blood from a newborn showing macrocytes and an occasional reticulocyte (×1000).

The red cells are macrocytic with an MCV ranging from 101 to 117 fL. The number of nucleated red cells ranges from 1 to 24 per 100 white blood cells. An occasional target cell, spherocyte and Howell Jolly body may be present. An occasional crenated cell may also be present, however this is an artefact and should not be included in the morphology report.

One-day-old neonate showing normal red cells for age.

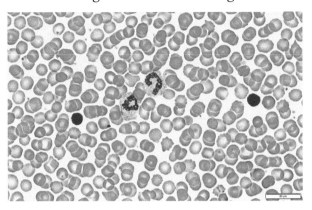

One-day-old neonate showing red cells normal for age (×1000).

Eight-year-old child showing red cells normal for age.

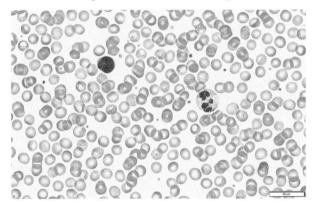

Eight-year-old child showing red cells normal for age (×1000).

Twelve-year-old child showing red cells normal for age.

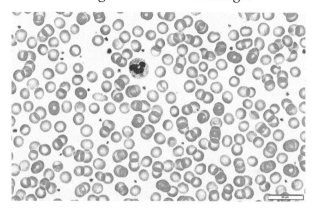

Twelve-year-old child showing red cells normal for age (×1000).

Iron deficiency anaemia showing fragmented red cells.

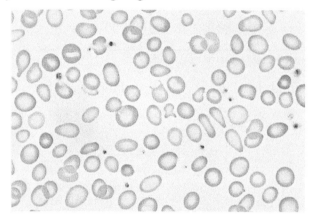

Iron deficiency anaemia showing a population of microcytic red cells as well as fragmented red cells (×1000).

Iron deficiency anaemia showing an increased number of elliptocytes.

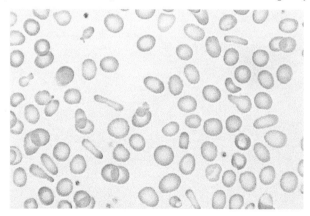

Iron deficiency anaemia showing an increased number of elliptocytes and pencil cells (×1000).

Two-year-old infant fed on cow's milk since birth showing a marked iron deficiency.

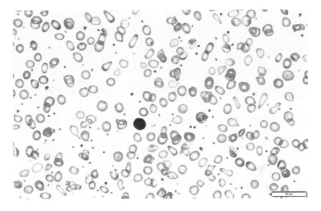

A two-year-old infant fed on cow's milk since birth showing a marked iron deficiency with a marked number of hypochromic microcytes and elliptocytes (×1000).

The above infant post transfusion showing a dimorphic blood film.

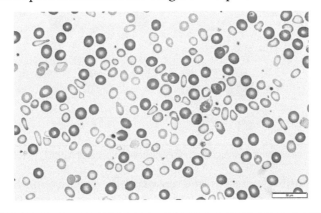

The above infant post transfusion showing a dimorphic blood film (×1000).

Anaemia in the neonate

ABO incompatibility

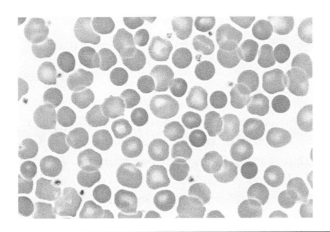

ABO incompatibility showing an increased number of spherocytes (×1000).

ABO haemolytic disease occurs most commonly in blood group O mothers and affects group A and B babies. The chief manifestation is jaundice within the first 24 hours of life. The haemoglobin concentration is usually normal.

The blood film shows increased numbers of spherocytes which stand out against a background of normochromic round macrocytes. The degree of polychromasia may be increased. The direct antiglobulin test (DAT) may be either negative or weakly positive.

Blood film showing an increased number of spherocytes.

Rh haemolytic disease of the newborn

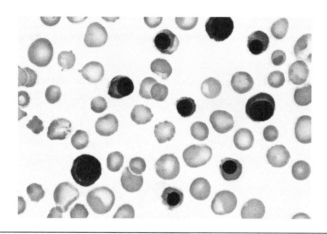

Rh haemolytic disease of the newborn showing an increased number of nucleated red cells (×1000).

When anti-D antibody present in a sensitised Rh-negative mother enters the fetal circulation, Rh-positive fetal cells are destroyed giving rise to a haemolytic process known as Rh haemolytic disease of the newborn.

This haemolytic process is characterised by jaundice with a low haemoglobin level (usually below 140 g/L) and a raised reticulocyte count (more than 7% and as high as 30–40%). There is an increase in the number of nucleated red blood cells per 100 white blood cells. The DAT is strongly positive. Spherocytes are usually not a feature of Rh haemolytic disease of the newborn.

Blood film showing an increased number of nucleated red cells.

Twin-to-twin haemorrhage prior to birth

Twin-to-twin haemorrhage occurs in monozygotic multiple pregnancies where there is a single placenta. The anaemic twin may have a Hb level as low as 35 g/L. It will be pale, weak and have cardiac failure. The polycythaemic twin may have a Hb level as high as 300 g/L. It develops the hyperviscosity syndrome. The anaemic twin can be transfused, however the polycythaemic twin is in trouble as it is virtually pumping treacle through its veins. Such a result should be notified to the clinician caring for the neonate *immediately*. Should the twin-to-twin haemorrhage be a gradual one there will be a significant difference in the birthweight of the twins.

The anaemic twin showing increased number of nucleated red blood cells (NRBCs) and reticulocytes.

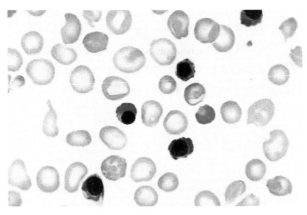

Twin-to-twin haemorrhage. The anaemic twin showing an increased number of nucleated red cells and raised reticulocyte count (×1000).

The polycythaemic twin showing an increased number of red cells and high Hb.

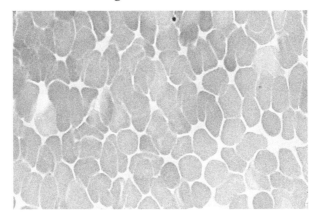

Twin-to-twin haemorrhage. The polycythaemic twin showing an increased number of red cells and high Hb (×1000).

Erythroblastosis fetalis

The following conditions can lead to erythroblastosis fetalis:

- Birth asphyxia
- Respiratory distress syndrome
- Pulmonary hypertension
- Meconium aspiration

The peripheral blood shows an increased number of NRBCs per 100 white blood cells (WBCs) together with a thrombocytopenia. The number of NRBCs can range from 500 to 800 per 100 WBCs.

The Hb and red cell count are usually normal in number. The reticulocyte count may be mildly elevated while the DAT is negative. A similar picture, together with thrombocytopenia, may be secondary to an intrauterine infection hence it may be necessary to perform a TORCH screen on the infant and on the mother. (TORCH: Toxoplasma, Others, Rubella, Cytomegalovirus and Herpes simplex.) This group of congenital infections can cause a neonatal thrombocytopenia.

Blood film showing anaemia and an increase in the number of NRBCs.

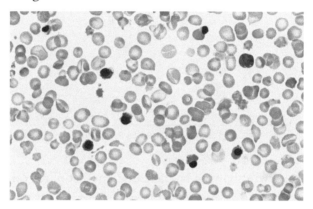

Erythroblastosis fetalis showing an increase in the number of nucleated red blood cells (×1000).

A second example also showing anaemia and an increase in the number of NRBCs.

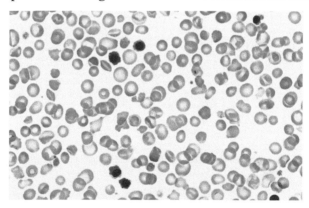

A second example of erythroblastosis fetalis showing anaemia and an increase in the number of nucleated red blood cells (×1000).

Haemoglobin disorders

The α-thalassaemias

The thalassaemias are hereditary anaemias that occur as a result of a mutation that affects the synthesis of normal haemoglobin. Normal haemoglobin consists of two pairs of dissimilar polypeptide chains, α-like and non-α (β, γ or δ). Each chain encloses an iron-containing porphyrin known as haem. The normal haemoglobins are:

- Haemoglobin A, consisting of two α- and two β-globin chains
- Haemoglobin A2, consisting of two α- and two δ-globin chains
- Haemoglobin F, consisting of two α- and two γ-globin chains

α-thalassaemia is characterised by a reduction or total lack of α-globin chains and β-thalassaemia by a reduction or total lack of β-globin genes. A microcytic hypochromic anaemia is associated with both α- and β-thalassaemia.

α-thalassaemia commonly occurs in populations from South-east Asia, the Mediterranean, Africa and China. It can arise when any number of four α-globin genes are either reduced or absent and hence can be divided into four groups.

Silent carrier α-thalassaemia trait
Silent carrier α-thalassaemia trait is characterised by minimal or no haematological changes. The haemoglobin level and the MCV are low normal. There is no obvious microcytosis seen on the blood film. The diagnosis of silent carrier α-thalassaemia is made by family studies and/or gene analysis.

α-thalassaemia trait

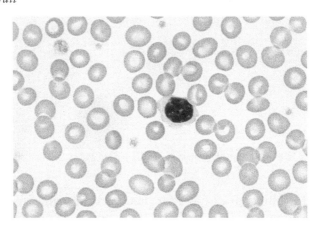

α-thalassaemia trait showing a microcytic hypochromic population of red cells (×1000).

This trait is characterised by a microcytic hypochromic blood film; the average MCV is 68 fL and the average MCH is 22 pg. HbH inclusion bodies (β4) are present after the blood is incubated at 37°C for 2 hours with a supra vital stain such as brilliant cresyl blue. The inclusion bodies represent precipitates of HbH and give the cell a golf ball-like appearance. Haemoglobin electrophoresis is normal in α-thalassaemia trait; thus, it is vital to detect the occasional HbH cell whose presence enables the diagnosis of α-thalassaemia trait to be made.

Haemoglobin H disease

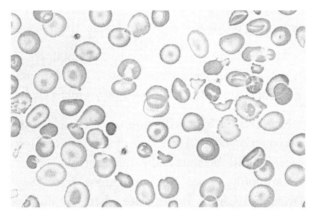

Haemoglobin H disease showing a markedly microcytic, hypochromic population of red cells with target cells and fragments (×1000).

Haemoglobin H disease cresyl blue

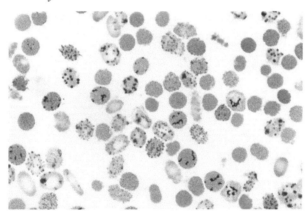

Haemoglobin H disease stained with a cresyl blue stain demonstrating the presence of HbH inclusions in the majority of the red cells (×1000).

Haemoglobin H (HbH) disease is characterised by a markedly microcytic hypochromic blood film with increased numbers of target cells and red cell fragments. The average MCV is 57 fL and the average MCH is 21 pg. HbH inclusions are present in the great majority of red cells.

Hydrops fetalis

Infants with hydrops fetalis are delivered stillborn at 30–40 weeks. The hydrops is due to a failure to produce α-globin genes. If a blood film can be obtained from the stillborn, it will show a characteristic population of large hypochromic macrocytes, marked polychromasia, basophilic stippling and increased numbers of nucleated red cells.

Haemoglobin constant spring (HbCS)

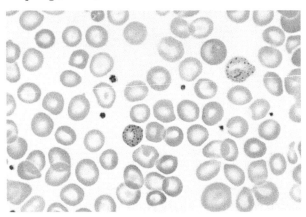

Haemoglobin constant spring showing coarse basophilic stippling in some of the red cells (×1000).

Haemoglobin H can be associated with a haemoglobin known as haemoglobin constant spring (HbCS). HbCS is an alpha chain variant rather than a deletion. The alpha chain is elongated by 31 additional amino acid residues at the C-terminal end making it very unstable. The presence of HbCS causes the red cells to break down faster than usual giving rise to a severe anaemia.

The red cells of HbCS are large and different from those seen in any of the other forms of thalassaemia. They are markedly overhydrated relative to those of the deletional forms of alpha thalassaemia. Coarse basophilic stippling is a characteristic feature of HbCS.

The *β*-thalassaemias

β-thalassaemia commonly occurs in populations of Mediterranean and African origin as well as in the Middle East, India and Pakistan, China and South-east Asia.

β-thalassaemia includes four syndromes: Silent carrier β-thalassaemia trait, β-thalassaemia trait, β-thalassaemia intermedia and β-thalassaemia major.

Silent carrier β-thalassaemia trait

Silent carrier β-thalassaemia trait is characterised by minimal or no haematological changes. The haemoglobin level and the MCV are low normal and there is no obvious microcytosis seen on the blood film. Characteristically, silent carriers of β-thalassaemia have normal levels of HbA_2. Diagnosis of silent carrier β-thalassaemia trait is made from family studies and/or gene analysis.

β–thalassaemia trait

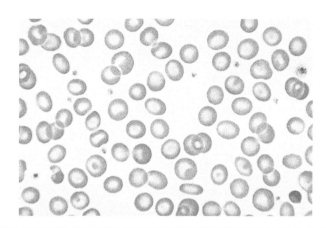

β-thalassaemia trait showing a microcytic, hypochromic population of red cells with target cells and fine basophilic stippling (×1000).

This trait is characterised by a microcytic hypochromic red cell picture together with target cells, elliptocytes and basophilic stippling. The average MCV is 63 fL and the average MCH is 20 pg.

In β-thalassaemia trait, the HbA2 level is increased above 3.5% and may be as high as 8.0%, while the HbF level is elevated in approximately 50% of patients, ranging from less than 1% to 5%.

β–thalassaemia intermedia

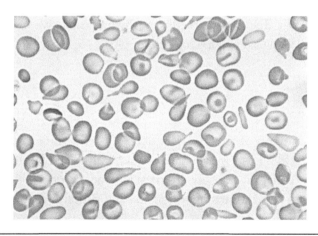

β-thalassaemia intermedia with a microcytic hyperchromic blood picture, teardrop poikilocytes and sometimes an occasional nucleated red blood cell (×1000).

This is a more severe form of β-thalassaemia trait but less severe than β-thalassaemia major. At the most severe end of the scale patients are transfusion dependent while at the less severe end they are transfusion independent. The red cell changes are more severe than those found in β-thalassaemia trait, with increased numbers of red cell poikilocytes. Teardrop poikilocytes are a prominent feature.

β–thalassaemia major

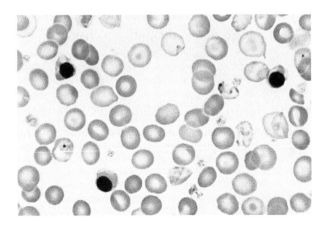

β-thalassaemia major: This is a case of β-thalassaemia major post splenectomy. It is microcytic hypochromic with Howell Jolly bodies, Pappenheimer bodies and nucleated red blood cells in a dimorphic blood film (×1000).

As the neonate has substantial HbF, anaemia in these patients usually develops during the first few months of life and becomes progressively worse in time. These infants will become transfusion dependent by the end of the first year of life; a later onset of the condition would suggest a case of thalassaemia intermedia.

β-thalassaemia major is characterised by Hb levels as low as 30 g/L and variable levels of HbF according to the transfusion status at the time of measurement. The acid elution or Kleihauer test shows that the HbF is evenly distributed among the red cells. The blood film shows a marked increase in the number of red cell poikilocytes namely, microcytosis and hypochromasia, target cells, basophilic stippling, Pappenheimer bodies (siderotic granules) and an increase in reticulocytes and nucleated red cells. As a result of frequent transfusions, the blood picture is often dimorphic and consequently the MCV and MCH are difficult to define.

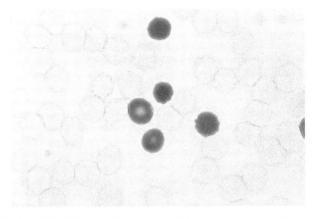

Kleihauer (acid-elution test) demonstrating the presence of HbF in fetal red cells. The cells containing adult haemoglobin appear as ghost cells (×1000).

Abnormal haemoglobins

Haemoglobin C, E and S (HbC, HbE and HbS) are abnormal haemoglobins characterised by an amino acid substitution in the β-globin chain.

Haemoglobin C

HbC ($\alpha_2\beta_2^{6Glu\rightarrow Lys}$) is an abnormal haemoglobin produced by the replacement of glutamic acid with lysine at the sixth position on the β chain. It is found in West Africans particularly from Ghana and the Upper Volta.

HbC trait

Individuals with HbC trait are clinically normal. Target cells are present in an otherwise normal blood film.

HbCC disease

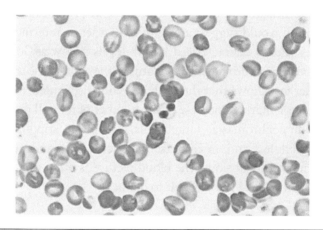

A case of haemoglobin CC (HbCC) showing some artefact target cells, however there is also a cell in the centre of the field containing two intraerythrocytic crystals present only in HbCC disease (×1000).

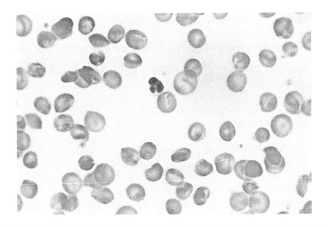

Another case of haemoglobin CC disease (×1000).

HbCC disease is associated with a haemolytic anaemia; the haemoglobin level ranges from 80 to 120 g/L. The blood film shows marked numbers of target cells, red cell fragments and microspherocytes. Upon careful examination, the red cells will be seen to contain intraerythrocytic crystals that dissolve readily when oxygen is released to the tissues. The MCV and MCH are slightly reduced as a result of the marked number of target cells that result from potassium efflux from the red cells, shrinking their contents with dehydration, leading to an increased ratio of surface area to volume.

In vitro test for detection of HbC

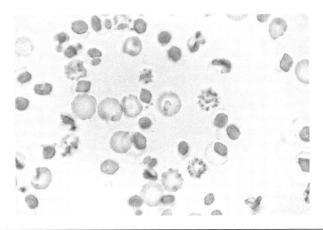

In vitro test for detection of haemoglobin C. Tetrahedral crystals in approximately 75% of the red cells (×1000).

An in vitro test to demonstrate the presence of HbC crystals may be performed by adding 3% NaCl to the red cells and examining a wet preparation under a coverslip after four hours or longer. Hypertonic dehydration of the red cells produces tetrahedral crystals in up to 75% of the red cells.

Haemoglobin E

HbE ($\alpha_2\beta_2^{26glu\rightarrow lys}$) is an abnormal haemoglobin produced by the replacement of glutamic acid with lysine at position 26 on the β chain. It is found in South-east Asians.

HbE trait

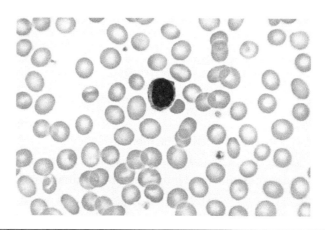

Haemoglobin E trait demonstrating a mild microcytic, hypochromic blood picture (×1000).

Individuals with HbE trait are asymptomatic, with haemoglobin levels of 120 g/L, average MCV of 74 fL and an average MCH of 25 pg. Occasional target cells may be present.

HbEE disease

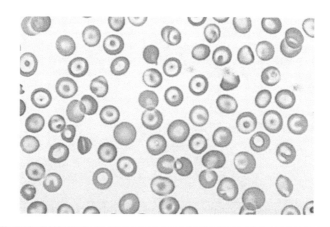

Haemoglobin EE disease demonstrating the presence of a marked number of target cells with a very low MCV and MCH and an absence of microcytes; classical of HbEE disease (×1000).

Haemoglobin EE (HbEE) disease is also asymptomatic; the haemoglobin level is rarely less than 100 g/L. The red cell indices are distinctly abnormal, with an average MCV of 58 fL and an average MCH of 20 pg. The red cell indices suggest a markedly microcytic and hypochromic blood film, with a marked number of target cells present. *NB Target cells have an increased surface area compared to volume, thus marked numbers of target cells will decrease the MCV and MCH.*

HbE/α thalassaemia

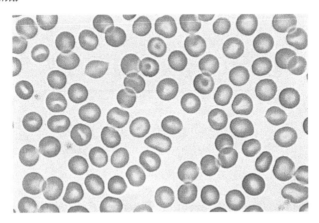

HbE/α thalassaemia (×1000).

HbE/β thalassaemia

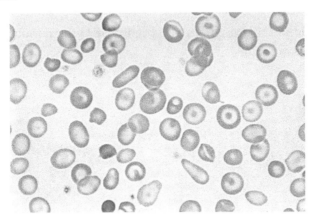

HbE/β thalassaemia (×1000).

HbS/β thalassaemia

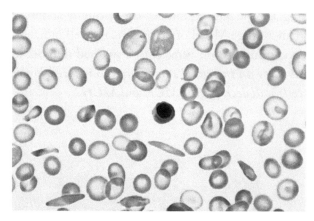

HbS/β thalassaemia (×1000).

Haemoglobin EPG required to diagnose all of the above.

Haemoglobin S

HbS ($\alpha_2\beta_2^{\,6glu\rightarrow val}$) is an abnormal haemoglobin produced by the replacement of glutamic acid with valine at the sixth position on the β chain and is found in the African as well as the American black population.

HbS trait

Individuals with HbS trait are clinically asymptomatic with normal haemoglobin levels and a normal blood film.

HbSS disease

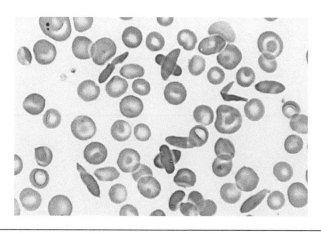

Haemoglobin SS disease characterised by the presence of moderate to marked number of sickle cells and an occasional Howell Jolly body (×1000).

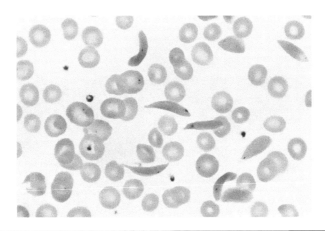

Haemoglobin SS disease showing the presence of Howell Jolly bodies (×1000).

Haemoglobin SS (HbSS) disease is charactered by a mild to moderate normo-chromic anaemia. The blood film shows a reticulocytosis with a varying number of sickle cells. Sickle cells are biconcave discs that, upon deoxygenation, change shape to become sickle shaped. Sickling is associated with the formation of liquid crystals of HbS that run parallel to the long axis of the cell and cause the sickle shape. When the cells containing HbS enter the fine capillaries of the body, they become deoxygenated, change shape and thus block off those capillaries. This process gives rise to small infarcts throughout the body especially in the spleen. As a result of this process, blood films of patients with sickle cell disease demonstrate features of autosplenectomy, namely Howell Jolly bodies, Pappenheimer bodies, target cells and nucleated red cells.

In vitro sickling test for detection of HbS

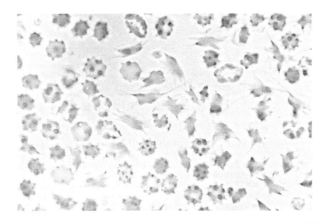

Haemoglobin S in vitro sodium dithionite preparation showing sickle cell test to demonstrate the presence of HbSS (×1000).

The reducing agent sodium dithionate induces red cells containing HbS to sickle. A mixture of red cells and sodium dithionate placed on a glass slide and sealed with a coverslip will reveal the presence of sickle-shaped cells within 1–12 hours.

Red cell membrane disorders

Hereditary spherocytosis

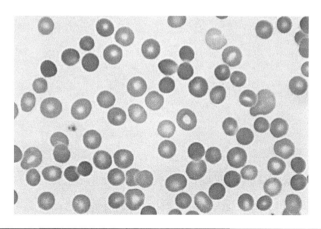

Hereditary spherocytosis demonstrating the presence of moderate spherocytes and an occasional polychromatic cell (×1000).

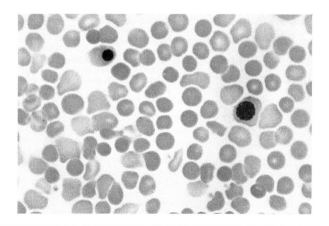

Hereditary spherocytosis in a newborn (×1000).

Spherocytes result from an intracorpuscular red cell membrane defect. Deficiency of spectrin, ankyrin or band 3 protein leads to the uncoupling of the skeletal lipid bilayer resulting in membrane loss in the form of microvesicles. This loss of surface area leads to the formation of spherocytes. The DAT will be negative while the degree of polychromasia will be increased. The eosin 5′ maleimide (EMA) binding by flow cytometry test will be reduced.

Note that hereditary spherocytosis can be diagnosed in neonates and very young infants by performing the eosin 5′ maleimide (EMA) test.

Hereditary elliptocytosis

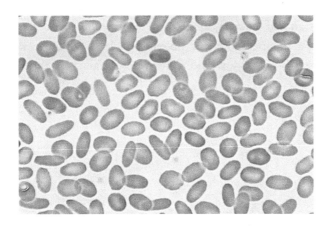

Hereditary elliptocytosis demonstrating 50 to 100% elliptocytes seen on routine blood film (×1000).

The elliptocytes of hereditary elliptocytosis (HE) demonstrate both quantitative and qualitative abnormalities in two major proteins comprising the membrane skeleton, namely spectrin and protein 4.1. There are various types of HE: The silent carrier, mild HE, HE associated with infantile hereditary pyropoikilocytosis and chronic haemolytic HE. Mild HE is the type that is commonly seen in the haematology laboratory. These patients usually have normal haemoglobin levels, but a mild compensated anaemia may be present. While approximately 5% of elliptocytes are seen on normal blood films, between 30 and 100% are seen on the blood film of mild HE.

South-east Asian ovalocytosis

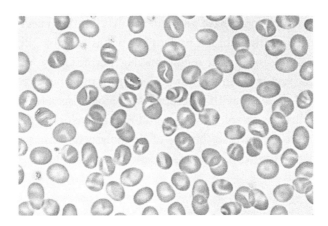

South-east Asian ovalocytosis: Peripheral blood showing oval-shaped stomatocytes, some with two transverse slits often 'v' and 'y' shaped slits. The mean cell volume is normal in this disorder (×1000).

This disorder is characterised by the presence of oval red cells, many of which contain one or two transverse bars or slits that give the cells the appearance of double stomatocytes. The slits can often appear as 'v' or 'y' shaped on the blood film. This abnormality results from increased ankyrin binding and decreased protein 3 mobility, leading to the production of rigid red cells. This rigidity acts as a protective mechanism against all strains of malaria, including *Plasmodium falciparum*. South-east Asian ovalocytosis is seen in up to 30% of people of Melanesian stock in Malaysia and Melanesia, particularly in the lowland tribes where malaria is endemic.

Hereditary stomatocytosis (hydrocytosis)

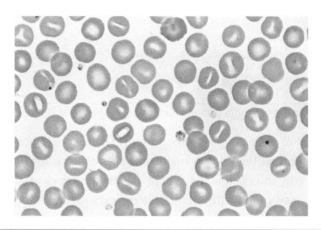

Hereditary stomatocytosis demonstrating the presence of macrocytes with a single slit and an occasional Howell Jolly body (post splenectomy) (×1000).

The Na⁺/K⁺ ATPase pump is greatly increased in hereditary stomatocytosis. The influx of Na^+ into red cells exceeds the loss of K^+ exiting the red cells. This leads to an increase in monovalent cation content causing the movement of water into the red cells. Hence the red cells swell and are transformed from discocytes to bowl forms. These bowl forms are known as stomatocytes and have an increased MCV. The defect in this disorder is due to the deficiency of a membrane protein known as protein 7.2b or stomatin. The function of this protein is to regulate membrane Na^+ permeability. Stomatocytes require increased energy to protect them against osmotic rupture. They are also vulnerable to splenic sequestration. Patients with hereditary stomatocytosis have a haemolytic anaemia. They are jaundiced with splenomegaly and often develop pigment gallstones later in life. Splenectomy may diminish the rate of haemolysis in these patients. Inheritance of hereditary stomatocytosis (hydrocytosis) is autosomal-dominant.

Hereditary xerocytosis

Hereditary xerocytosis is a rare autosomal-dominant haemolytic anaemia. The red cells are dehydrated as there is a loss of potassium exiting the cell compared with the amount of sodium entering the cell. Thus, the intracellular cation content and water content are reduced. The enzyme involved in the passage of anions across the red cell membrane, glyceraldehyde-3-phosphate dehydrogenase, is increased. The blood picture is that of a severe haemolytic anaemia. The MCV may be slightly increased due to the presence of increased reticulocytes. Target cells are prominent and there may be some 'puddling' of haemoglobin towards the periphery of the red cells.

Hereditary pyropoikilocytosis (HPP)

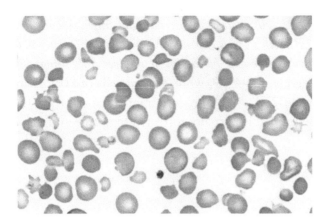

Hereditary pyropoikilocytosis characterised by extreme poikilocytes, red cell budding, triangular fragments, spherocytes and elliptocytes. Also note low MCV in newborn (×1000).

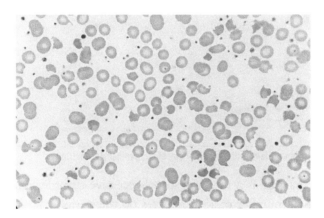

Hereditary pyropoikilocytosis in a 15-day-old infant (×1000). (Courtesy of Ethné van der Heyde, Red Cross Children's Hospital, Cape Town, South Africa.)

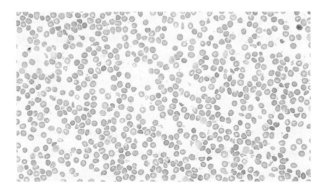

Hereditary pyropoikilocytosis in a five-week-old infant (×1000).

Hereditary pyropoikilocytosis (HPP) presents at birth and persists into infancy. It is characterised by the presence of extreme poikilocytosis with red cell budding, triangular fragments, spherocytes and elliptocytes. The MCV is significantly reduced owing to the presence of large numbers of triangular fragments. *Whereas the MCV at birth in a non-affected neonate ranges from 101 to 117 fL, the MCV in a neonate with HPP will be in the mid-80 fL. Also note that the triangular fragments are TRUE fragments and should not be reported as schistocytes. The number of red cell fragments reduces over time with the majority of red cells seen on the blood film in an older child being elliptocytes.* Note that normal red cells fragment at 49°C, while the red cells of HPP fragment at 45–46°C. Prolonged heating at 37°C will also induce fragmentation; thus, these patients suffer from a severe anaemia that is partially corrected by splenectomy.

Abetalipoproteinaemia

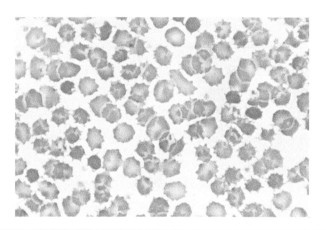

Abetalipoproteinaemia: Newborn infant with a marked number of acanthocytes (×1000).

Abetalipoproteinaemia is a rare autosomal-recessive disorder characterised by the presence of a marked number of acanthocytes on the peripheral blood film. The primary defect is due to a mutation and lack of activity in the microsomal triglyceride transfer protein needed to bind lipids to the β-apolipoprotein in plasma. The plasma triglycerides are almost absent and the plasma cholesterol is markedly decreased. There is an increase in sphingomyelin in the outer half of the red cell membrane bilayer, increasing the surface layer of the cell. This β-apolipoprotein defect leads to the production of acanthocytes, about 50–90% of the red cells are acanthocytes. The sphingomyelin accumulates with cell ageing; hence the nucleated precursor red cells and the reticulocytes are not affected.

Abetalipoproteinaemia is characterised clinically by ataxic neurologic disease, retinitis pigmentosa (often leading to blindness) and fat malabsorption. The neurologic abnormalities present between five and ten years of age and continue until death in the second to third decade. Despite the marked number of acanthocytes seen in these patients, anaemia and haemolysis is not a feature of this disorder. The haemoglobin levels are normal.

Vitamin E deficiency

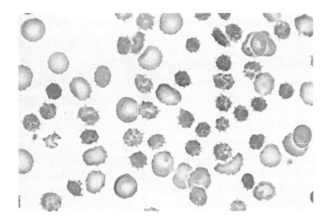

Vitamin E deficiency: Showing a population of red cells resembling spur cells at about 4–6 weeks of life (×1000).

Vitamin E (α-tocopherol) is a fat-soluble vitamin that appears to serve as an antioxidant in humans. Nutritional deficiency of vitamin E is extremely rare as α-tocopherol occurs in many food products and the daily requirement is only 5–7 mg. Vitamin E deficiency in humans is virtually limited to the neonatal period and to pathologic states associated with chronic fat malabsorption. Low-birth-weight infants are born with low serum and tissue concentrations of vitamin E. When these infants are fed a diet unusually rich in polyunsaturated fatty acids and inadequate vitamin E, a haemolytic anaemia will develop by 4–6 weeks of age. The anaemia is associated with morphologic alterations of the red cell membrane. A haemolytic anaemia due to increased splenic sequestration follows. Treatment with vitamin E produces a prompt reversal of this process. Modifications of infant formulas have all but eliminated vitamin E deficiency in the preterm infant.

Liver disease

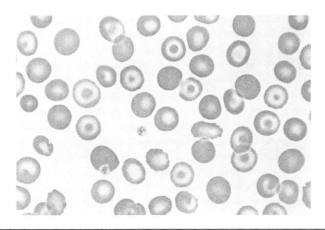

Liver disease: Round macrocytes and target cells (×1000).

Obstructive liver disease is characterised by the presence of target cells and round macrocytes. Target cells have a characteristic distribution of haemoglobin in the centre of the cell as well as around the periphery. The ratio of surface area to volume is greater than normal since the red cell membrane is expanded by the accumulation of lecithin and cholesterol from free exchange with plasma lipids. In obstructive jaundice and hepatitis with biliary obstruction, there is an increase of free cholesterol and lecithin in the plasma due to the bile salts that inhibit the activity of the enzyme lecithin-cholesterol acyl transferase, which normally esterifies cholesterol.

Burns – (third degree)

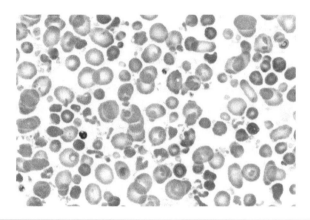

Third-degree burns: Red cell budding, fragments, microcytes and microspherocytes. False high platelet count (×1000).

Third-degree burns induce changes on the blood film that can be seen almost immediately after the event. Direct action of heat at 49°C denatures spectrin in the red cell membrane, giving rise to red cell budding, fragmentation, microcytes and microspherocytes. The presence of the above changes falsely elevates the platelet count, hence the need for a manual count where possible.

Diamond–Blackfan anaemia (DBA)

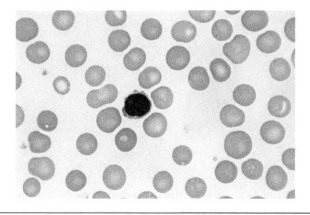

Diamond–Blackfan anaemia: Anaemia, reticulocytopenia; red cells macrocytic for age (×1000).

Diamond–Blackfan anaemia (DBA) is a congenital pure red cell aplasia diagnosed in children usually less than one year of age. Craniofacial abnormalities are associated with DBA. These include a flat nasal bridge, wide-set eyes and a thick upper lip as well as deafness and short stature. The haemoglobin levels at birth have a mean value of 70 g/L and can be as low as 26 g/L. The red cells are invariably macrocytic for age. A reticulocytopenia is present. The bone marrow shows erythroid hypoplasia. The myeloid cells and megakaryocytes are normal in number while the lymphocytes are increased in number.

Haemolytic anaemias

Haemolytic anaemia due to lead poisoning

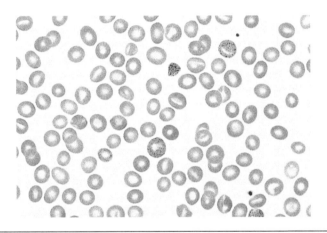

Lead poisoning: Coarse, basophilic stippling in the red cells (×1000).

The ingestion of lead interferes with haem synthesis. It does so by inhibiting several of the enzymes directly involved with haem synthesis. Pyrimidine 5′-nucleotidase is one such enzyme. In its absence pyrimidine nucleotides accumulate in the red cells, preventing iron from being incorporated into haem at a normal rate. This leads to a shortened red cell lifespan resulting in a mild haemolytic anaemia. The blood film shows characteristic fine to coarse basophilic stippling in the red cells as seen with any of the Romanowsky stains. The anticoagulant ethylene diamine tetra-acetic acid (EDTA) can mask lead-induced stippling if blood films are not made fresh and fixed in methanol immediately.

Oxidant-drug-induced haemolytic anaemia

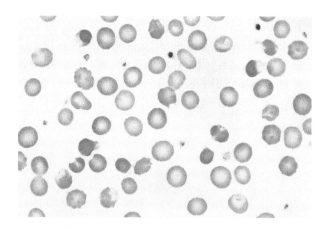

Note the presence of bite cells and blister cells. Be mindful of the fact that spherocytes are NOT a feature of oxidant hae-molysis (×1000).

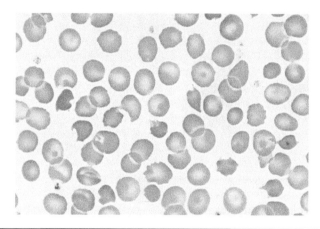

Oxidant haemolysis in a newborn probably due to naphthalene (moth balls). The red cells which are macrocytic for age and demonstrate the presence of bite cells (×1000).

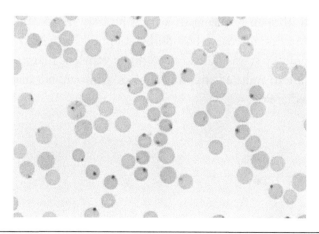

Heinz bodies: Cresyl blue stain (supra vital stain) demonstrating the presence of Heinz bodies (×1000).

The use of oxidant drugs can be easily recognised from the blood film, provided that the patient has not had a splenectomy. Two frequently used oxidant drugs, dapsone and sulfasalazine (Salazopyrin) as well as the antibiotic Bactrim may induce a Heinz-body-positive haemolytic anaemia resulting in a blood picture characterised by the presence of bite and blister cells should the patient be G6PD deficient. Heinz bodies are precipitates of denatured haemoglobin and are the manifestation of the oxidative challenge that the red cell has suffered. They are rapidly removed or pitted out by the spleen, giving rise to bite cells. Should the red cell membrane of the bite cell re-join, a blister cell will result. The red cells of premature infants and neonates are more susceptible to oxidants. Prolonged exposure to naphthalene may give rise to a haemolytic anaemia in infants despite normal levels of the enzyme glucose-6-phosphate dehydrogenase (G6PD). Also, the consumption of fava beans in young children who are G6PD deficient will give rise to oxidant haemolysis.

In the case of G6PD deficiency, when a G6PD assay has been requested, the scientist must ensure that the haemoglobin level and the reticulocyte count have both returned to normal before blood is collected. Reticulocytes have an increased level of G6PD thus can falsely increase the result.

Pyruvate kinase (PK) deficiency

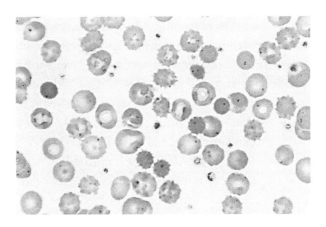

Blood film from a case of pyruvate kinase deficiency post splenectomy demonstrating the presence of Howell Jolly bodies, Pappenheimer bodies and prickle cells (×1000).

Pyruvate kinase (PK) is an erythrocyte glycolytic enzyme involved in the Embden–Myerhoff pathway of metabolism. Deficiency of this enzyme is associated with chronic haemolysis and thus anaemia, jaundice and splenomegaly. In some cases the anaemia may be profound, presenting in early infancy and requiring frequent blood transfusions. In other cases, the anaemia may be so mild that the deficiency may not be discovered until late childhood or even adulthood.

The blood film shows a red cell picture consistent with that of a haemolytic anaemia with an occasional prickle cell. The number of prickle cells is strikingly increased together with Howell Jolly bodies and Pappenheimer bodies following splenectomy.

Autoimmune haemolytic anaemia (AIHA)

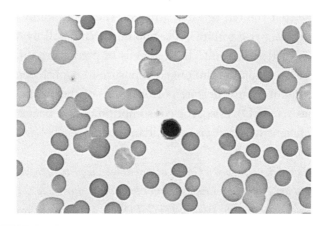

Autoimmune haemolytic anaemia: This blood film shows the presence of a wide-thermal-amplitude auto-antibody giving rise to features of both a warm and cold autoimmune haemolytic anaemia. Note the presence of spherocytes, polychromasia and auto-agglutination (×1000).

Autoimmune haemolytic anaemia (AIHA) is due to antibodies produced by the body's immune system against its own cells. These antibodies are either warm or cold and in some instances may have a wide thermal amplitude extending from warm to cold. Warm antibody AIHA is the most common type; the antibodies produced are of the IgG class, which have maximal activity at 37°C. Cold antibody AIHA results from the production of antibodies of the IgM class, which act at temperatures below 37°C. Examination of the blood film from a case of AIHA reveals the presence of spherocytes, polychromasia and nucleated red cells. In cold AIHA, auto-agglutination will also be present. The diagnosis of AIHA is established by performing a DAT on the patient's red cells. A positive result indicates the presence of antibody or complement on the red cell surface, thus confirming the diagnosis of AIHA.

The DAT can also be used to differentiate AIHA from hereditary spherocytosis (HS): both disorders have a similar blood picture but the red cells in HS result from an intracorpuscular red cell membrane defect and are thus DAT negative while the red cells in AIHA will be DAT positive.

Microangiopathic haemolytic anaemia

The term 'microangiopathic' means small vessel disease; hence microangiopathic haemolytic anaemia results from physical damage to red cells as they pass through very small orifices or damaged and sclerosed vessels. The blood film shows increased numbers of red cell fragments that have characteristically sharp projections. *These fragments are referred to as schistocytes, red cells produced by a microangiopathic process. They are fractured or ripped as they pass across strands of fibrin in damaged vessels or as they pass across a damaged or prosthetic heart valve.* Thrombocytopenia is a classical finding in some types of microangiopathic haemolytic anaemia. A variety of disorders is associated with a microangiopathic blood picture, namely haemolytic uraemic syndrome (HUS), thrombotic thrombocytopenic purpura (TTP), human immunodeficiency virus (HIV) infection, disseminated intravascular coagulation (DIC), valvular heart disease, HELLP or preeclampsia of pregnancy, necrotising enterocolitis (NEC), Marfan's syndrome, malignancy and acute renal failure. Microangiopathic haemolytic anaemia may also result from the use of the immunosuppressive agent Cyclosporin.

Valvular heart disease

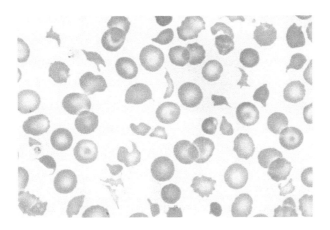

Microangiopathic haemolytic anaemia: A case of valvular heart disease or mechanical haemolysis showing the presence of schistocytes, sharp pointed fragments which have been sheared off and must be referred to as 'schistocytes.' The platelet count is within the normal range in this case (×1000).

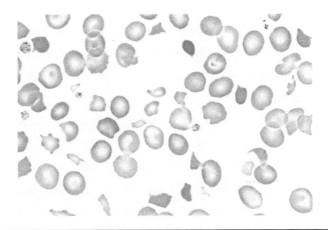

A second case as above indicating the same features (×1000).

Microangiopathic haemolytic anaemia occurs in valvular heart disease and also in some patients who have prosthetic heart valves inserted. The high shear forces produced by the abnormal blood flow seen in such disorders produce a blood film characterised by the presence of *schistocytes*, classical of a microangiopathic process. The platelet count is invariably normal.

Haemolytic uraemic syndrome (HUS)

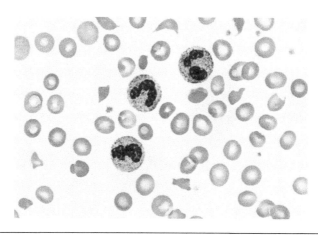

Haemolytic uraemic syndrome in a two-year-old child showing the presence of an absolute neutrophilia with hypergranulated neutrophils together with schistocytes (×1000).

Haemolytic uraemic syndrome (HUS) occurs most commonly in infancy and early childhood and is initiated by infection with *Escherichia coli* strain 0157. This bacterium produces a verocytotoxin that is attracted to the vascular endothelium lining the glomeruli of the kidney. This toxin induces severe glomerulonephritis that in turn leads to a microangiopathic blood picture.

Thrombotic thrombocytopenic purpura (TTP)

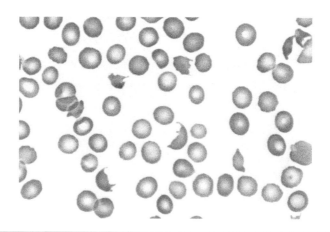

Thrombotic thrombocytopenic purpura: Peripheral blood film showing schistocytes and thrombocytopenia (×1000).

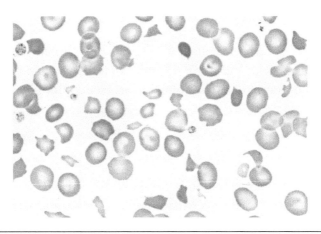

Necrotising enterocolitis in a premature newborn showing the presence of schistocytes and thrombocytopenia (×1000).

Thrombotic thrombocytopenic purpura (TTP) is a microangiopathic haemolytic anaemia seen mostly in adults. It is characterised by a pentad of clinical features, namely fever, thrombocytopenia, anaemia, neurological symptoms and renal disease; schistocytes are seen on the blood film. TTP has been reported in patients with the acquired immunodeficiency syndrome (AIDS)-related complex.

Marfan's syndrome

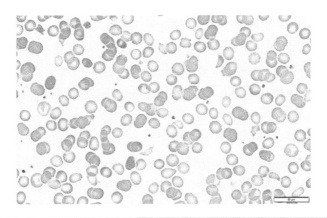

Marfan's syndrome showing the presence of schistocytes on the blood film (×1000).

Marfan's syndrome is a multi-systemic genetic disorder that affects the connective tissue, especially in the heart. Patients with Marfan's syndrome tend to be tall and thin, with long arms, legs, fingers and toes. The most serious complication of Marfan's syndrome involves the aorta, with an increased risk of mitral valve prolapse and aortic aneurysm. Aortic dissection occurs when a small tear occurs between the inner and outer layer of the aorta allowing blood to squeeze between the two layers giving rise to the presence of schistocytes on the blood film.

Disseminated intravascular coagulation (DIC)

Disseminated intravascular coagulation (DIC) occurs when small blood vessels become blocked by platelet and fibrin thrombi, thus altering the patency of the vessel and inducing intravascular haemolysis. The blood film shows *schistocytes* and thrombocytopenia.

Malignancy

A microangiopathic haemolytic anaemia may be associated with metastatic carcinoma, especially mucin-secreting adenocarcinoma of the breast and stomach. Metastases occurring in the microvascular system, especially the lung, give rise to a microangiopathic blood picture with thrombocytopenia.

HELLP syndrome

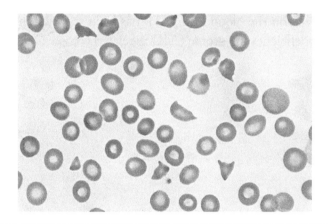

HELLP syndrome showing the presence of schistocytes (×1000).

The HELLP syndrome (haemolysis, elevated liver enzymes and low platelet count) is a multisystem syndrome occurring in preeclampsia and eclampsia. It affects both primiparous and multiparous women in the third trimester of pregnancy. HELLP is characterised by a microangiopathic haemolytic anaemia, *schistocytes*, hepatic dysfunction and renal failure, and in severe cases, DIC.

Delivery of the fetus is the initial treatment; however, the disease remains active after delivery and appears to achieve peak intensity during the 24–48-hour post-delivery period.

Paroxysmal cold haemoglobinuria (PCH)

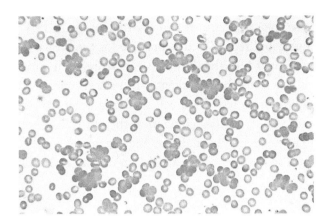

Paroxysmal cold haemoglobinuria. Donath–Landsteiner antibody positive haemolytic anaemia. Peripheral blood film showing auto-agglutination, spherocytes and reticulocytes (×400).

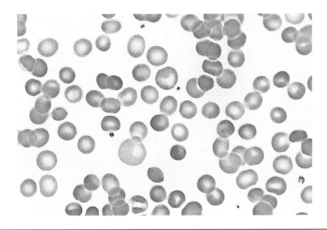

Paroxysmal cold haemoglobinuria showing auto-agglutination, spherocytes and reticulocytes (×1000).

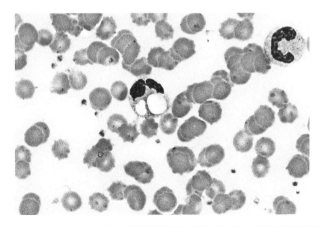

Paroxysmal cold haemoglobinuria showing granulocytic erythrophagocytosis (×1000).

Paroxysmal cold haemoglobinuria (PCH) is an autoimmune haemolytic anaemia described by Julius Donath and Karl Landsteiner in 1904. It occurs in children under five years of age. The blood picture resembles that of an AIHA with spherocytes, reticulocytes and nucleated red cells. It is positive for the Donath–Landsteiner antibody which is a polyclonal IgG that binds to various red cell antigens such as I, i, P and p on the red cell surface. The P antigen is its primary target. The polyclonal IgG anti-P autoantibody binds to red blood cell surface antigens in the cold. When the blood returns to the warmer central circulation the red cells are lysed with complement, giving rise to intravascular haemolysis. The anaemia is DAT (C3d) positive. The blood film sometimes shows monocytic and granulocytic erythrophagocytosis.

Congenital sideroblastic anaemia

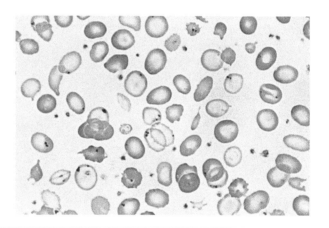

Congenital sideroblastic anaemia showing a dimorphic blood picture (transfusion dependent) with many Pappenheimer bodies (×1000).

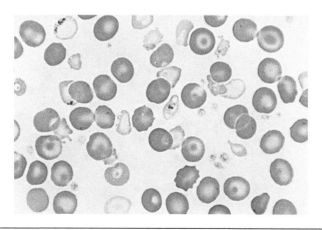

Congenital sideroblastic anaemia showing a marked dimorphic blood picture with Pappenheimer bodies (×1000).

Presents in early childhood mainly in males and is characterised by a dimorphic blood picture. The bone marrow is hypercellular with erythroid hyperplasia. Some of the erythroblasts show microerythroblastic as well as defective haemoglobinisation with ragged and vacuolated cytoplasm. When the film is stained with a Perl's Prussian blue stain ringed sideroblasts will be evident. Ringed sideroblasts represent the presence of perinuclear mitochondria containing large deposits of inorganic iron. Haem production is impaired and there is ineffective erythropoiesis. Iron stores are increased.

Transient erythroblastopenia of childhood (TEC)

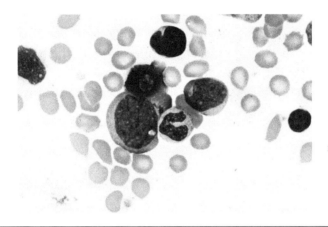

Parvovirus B19 infection: Bone marrow from a seven-month-old child showing the presence of a giant proerythroblast (×1000).

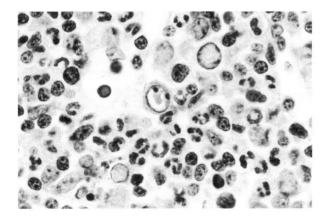

Parvovirus B19 infection. Bone marrow trephine showing an intracellular viral inclusion within a giant proerythroblast (×1000).

Transient erythroblastopenia of childhood (TEC) is an acquired red cell aplasia occurring in previously healthy children usually between the ages of one and three years. It is frequently preceded by a viral infection some two months prior to presentation. TEC is a self-limiting disease with patients often presenting during the recovery phase of the infection. The platelet count is normal except in those cases preceded by a viral infection such as parvovirus B19 infection, where the count may be significantly reduced.

The bone marrow shows erythroid hypoplasia. There is often a maturation arrest in the erythroid lineage. Should the bone marrow be sampled during the recovery phase, erythropoiesis will be markedly increased. Spontaneous and complete recovery usually occurs within two months of diagnosis.

Infection with parvovirus B19 may lead to TEC in a variety of genetically inherited anaemias such as hereditary spherocytosis, PK deficiency, sickle cell disease, autoimmune haemolytic anaemia and thalassaemia. Parvovirus B19 may also cause thrombocytopenia and/or neutropenia in otherwise healthy children.

The virus infects the erythroid progenitors using the P antigen as a receptor, preventing replication and maturation of the infected cell. The bone marrow in these infected patients shows a relative absence of erythroid precursors as well as the presence of giant proerythroblasts. The aplasia is transient and the marrow recovers usually within one to two weeks.

Recovery from TEC

Recovery is denoted by a rise in the reticulocyte count and a reversal of the neutropenia. Spontaneous, complete recovery usually occurs within one month of presentation. There is no specific treatment for TEC; the administration of intravenous IgG or corticosteroids is not indicated.

Miscellaneous red cell images

Splenectomy – Howell Jolly bodies

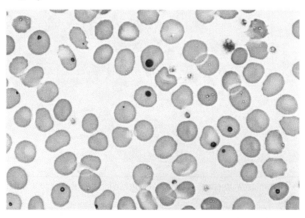

Post splenectomy blood film showing a marked number of Howell Jolly bodies (×1000).

Splenectomy – Acanthocytes

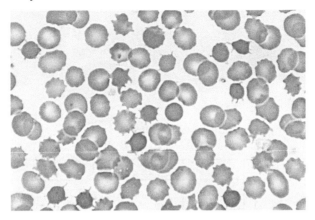

Post splenectomy blood film showing a marked number of acanthocytes (×1000).

Lipaemic plasma

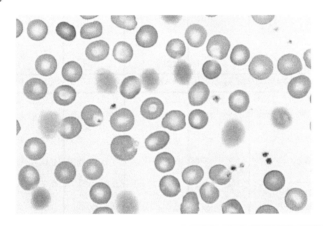

Hyperlipidaemia: Blood film showing the presence of ghost cells with an indistinct red cell membrane (×1000).

White cell reference ranges in infancy and childhood

AGE	WCC(x10⁹/L)		N(%)		L(%)		M(%)		E(%)		B(%)	
0-1 d	9.6	30.4	39	73	13	47	4	15	0	7	0	2
1-7 d	7.5	21.0	20	73	30	70	4	15	0	7	0	2
1-2 w	6.8	20.0	15	60	35	75	4	15	0	7	0	2
2w – 3m	6.4	12.1	11	44	40	80	4	12	1	7	0	2
3-6 m	5.6	14.1	7	35	53	83	3	14	0	6	0	1
6m – 2y	5.4	13.6	14	55	37	79	2	12	0	6	0	1
2-4 y	4.9	12.8	24	67	28	64	2	11	0	7	0	1
4-8 y	4.7	12.3	32	71	20	59	2	10	0	8	0	1
8-12 y	4.7	12.2	37	70	22	55	2	10	1	8	0	1

AGE	N(A) x10⁹/L		L(A) x10⁹/L		M(A) x10⁹/L		E(A) x10⁹/L		B(A) x10⁹/L		NRBC	
0-1 d	4.4	21.0	2.5	9.1	0.6	4.1	0.0	1.3	0.0	0.4	1	24
1-7 d	1.5	15.3	2.3	14.7	0.3	1.5	0.1	1.3	0.0	0.4		
1-2 w	1.0	12.0	2.4	15.0	0.3	1.5	0.1	1.3	0.0	0.4		
2w – 3m	0.8	4.9	3.8	7.6	0.3	1.2	0.1	0.8	0.0	0.2		
3-6 m	0.5	4.4	3.4	9.8	0.2	1.1	0.0	0.7	0.0	0.1		
6m – 2y	1.1	6.0	2.7	8.9	0.2	1.1	0.0	0.6	0.0	0.1		
2-4 y	1.7	6.7	2.0	6.6	0.2	1.0	0.0	0.6	0.0	0.1		
4-8 y	1.8	7.7	1.6	5.1	0.1	1.0	0.0	0.6	0.0	0.1		
8-12 y	1.8	7.6	1.7	4.5	0.2	0.9	0.1	0.6	0.0	0.1		

This chart demonstrates reference ranges for white cells from 0–1 day (cord blood) to 12 years of age (puberty).

This chart demonstrates both the percentage and absolute counts of neutrophils, lymphocytes, monocytes, eosinophils and basophils ranging in age from 0–1 day to 12 years of age. Also note the nucleated red cell count (NRBC) ranges from 1 to 24 NRBCs at birth.

DOI: 10.1201/9781003474432-3

AGE	N(A) x10⁹/L		L(A) x10⁹/L	
0-1 d	4.4	21.0	2.5	9.1
1-7 d	1.5	15.3	2.3	14.7
1-2 w	1.0	12.0	2.4	15.0
2w – 3m	0.8	4.9	3.8	7.6
3-6 m	0.5	4.4	3.4	9.8
6m – 2y	1.1	6.0	2.7	8.9
2-4 y	1.7	6.7	2.0	6.6
4-8 y	1.8	7.7	1.6	5.1
8-12 y	1.8	7.6	1.7	4.5

This is a simplified chart emphasising the absolute neutrophil and lymphocyte counts ranging from 0–1 day to 12 years of age.

This is a simplified chart emphasising the absolute neutrophil count $\times10^9$/L versus the absolute lymphocyte count $\times10^9$/L ranging from 0–1 day to 12 years of age.

Myeloid maturation

The earliest recognisable cell in the myeloid lineage is the myeloblast. This gives rise sequentially to the promyelocyte, myelocyte, metamyelocyte, band form and neutrophil, eosinophil and basophil.

Myeloblast

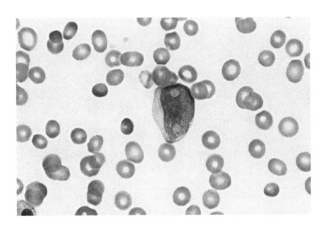

Myeloblast (×1000).

The myeloblast varies in size from 15 to 20 μm in diameter: It has a round nucleus occupying approximately 80% of the cell. The chromatin is fine with one to three nucleoli. The cytoplasm is basophilic in colour and agranular.

Promyelocyte

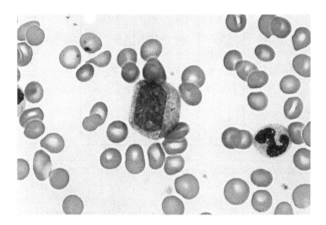

Promyelocyte (×1000).

The promyelocyte is the next stage in the maturation process. It is also approximately 15–20 μm in diameter. The chromatin is denser and also contains nucleoli. The cytoplasm is still basophilic but contains fine azurophilic or primary granules.

Myelocyte

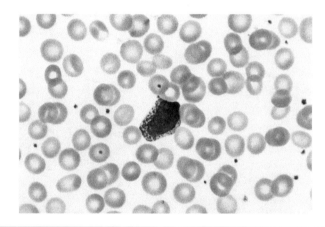

Early myelocyte (×1000).

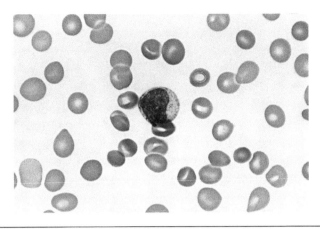

Late myelocyte (×1000).

The myelocyte may be up to 25 μm in diameter. There are no nucleoli present while the chromatin pattern is again denser. The nucleus to cytoplasmic ratio (N/C) is decreased. Primary granules may be seen in the early myelocyte while the late myelocyte or more developed myelocyte contains specific or secondary granules. The composition of these secondary granules determines whether the myelocyte will develop into a neutrophil, an eosinophil or a basophil.

Metamyelocyte

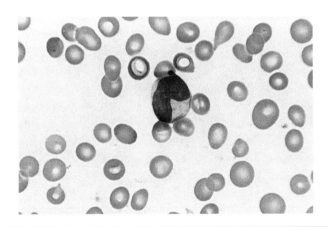

Metamyelocyte (×1000).

The metamyelocyte ranges in size between 10 and 18 μm. It is characterised by the presence of an indented nucleus resembling the shape of a broad bean. The chromatin pattern is thicker and more densely staining than the myelocyte while the cytoplasm contains many fine specific granules.

Band form

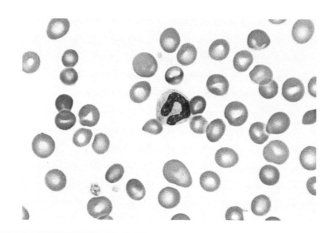

Band form (×1000).

The band form ranges in size from 10 to 15 μm. It has a deeply indented U-shaped nucleus composed of coarsely clumped chromatin. The cytoplasm is pink and contains many specific pink granules.

Neutrophil

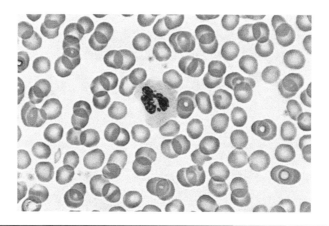

Neutrophil (×1000).

The neutrophil is the most mature stage in the myeloid series (together with the eosinophil and the basophil). The neutrophil is approximately 12–14 μm in diameter. The nucleus is lobulated with three to four lobes connected by thin strands of chromatin. The cytoplasm is pink and contains specific granules. A morphological difference between neutrophils of males and females is that female neutrophils have an appendage shaped like a drumstick. These appendages are attached to one lobe of the nucleus by a thin strand of chromatin. Neutrophils have phagocytic properties.

Eosinophil

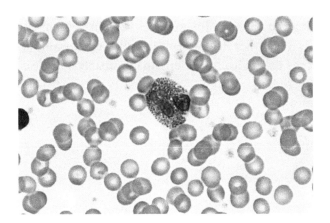

Eosinophil (×1000).

The eosinophil develops through the same stages as the neutrophil, the specific eosinophil granules first appearing at the myelocyte stage. The eosinophilic myelocyte, metamyelocyte and band form have the same structural characteristics as their neutrophilic counterparts. The mature eosinophil is a round cell 12–17 μm in diameter and is a phagocytic cell (although less so than the neutrophil). It is characterised by the presence of large round granules with an affinity for acid dyes such as eosin. The nucleus has two to three lobes. Eosinophils are attracted to sites of antigen-antibody interaction in tissues, especially in cases of foreign protein sensitisation such as allergic disorders and parasitic infections.

Basophil

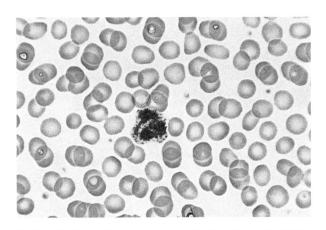

Basophil (×1000).

The basophil develops through the same stages as the neutrophil and the eosinophil. Similarly, the specific granules appear at the myelocyte stage. The basophil is a round cell approximately 10–14 μm in diameter with a bilobed nucleus. The granules are large and bluish black in colour and are present in the cytoplasm as well as overlying and partly obscuring the nucleus. The granules contain heparin and histamine. Their phagocytic power is weak; they degranulate and release histamine at sites of inflammation or when allergens react with IgE. Heparin is probably not released from basophils.

Abnormal myeloid cells

Pelger–Huët anomaly

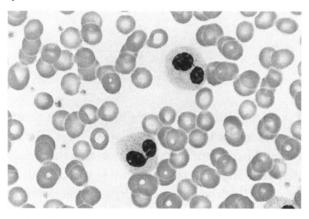

Pelger–Huët anomaly showing classical 'spectacle form' nuclei (×1000).

This is a congenital anomaly. In the heterozygous form, the neutrophils have one or two nuclear lobes. The chromatin pattern is dense and pyknotic. Often the lobes are joined by a fine strand of chromatin giving the appearance of spectacles. In the homozygous form, the neutrophils contain only single, round nuclei with a dense chromatin pattern.

Hypersegmented neutrophil

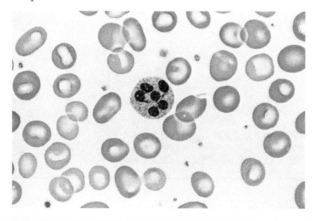

Hypersegmented neutrophil (×1000).

A hypersegmented neutrophil is one in which the nucleus has six or more lobes. An increased number of hypersegmented neutrophils is found in megaloblastic anaemia and following antimetabolite cytotoxic therapy. Should there be an increased number of neutrophils observed with five lobes the comment 'hypersegmented' neutrophils should also be reported.

Hypergranulated neutrophils

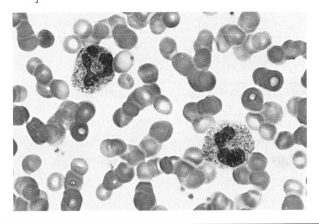

Hypergranular neutrophils (×1000).

When the presence of blue-black granules are noted within the cytoplasm of neutrophils it should be reported as 'hypergranulated' neutrophils. Such granules are azurophilic granules that are present when the neutrophil is activated secondary to the presence of a bacterial infection or a toxic state. Also note that such granules will also be present secondary to the administration of cytokines such as granulocyte colony stimulating factor (G-CSF) or granulocyte macrophage colony stimulating factor (GM-CSF) therapy. Granules with the same appearance will also be observed in Alder Reilly anomaly. *Thus, the statement 'toxic' should be used judiciously. Always consider the clinical notes before reporting on 'toxic neutrophils.'*

Toxic vacuolation

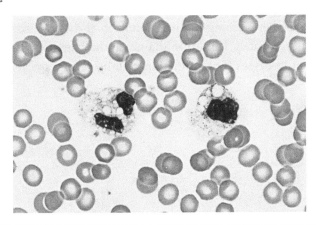

Toxic vacuolation in the neutrophils resulting from a bacterial infection (×1000).

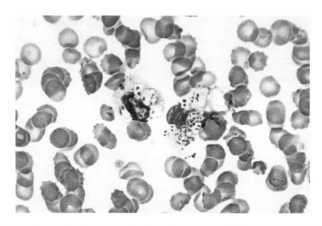

Toxic vacuolation showing phagocytosed bacteria in a case of severe septicaemia (×1000).

Toxic vacuolation is commonly seen in the cytoplasm of neutrophils containing toxic granules. These vacuoles, known as phagocytic vacuoles, often contain phagocytosed bacteria. Vacuolation can also be induced in neutrophils that have been stored in EDTA for more than 24 hours.

Döhle bodies

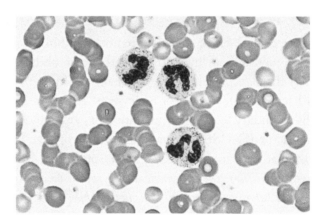

Döhle bodies in the cytoplasm of septic neutrophils (×1000).

Döhle bodies are blue-staining bodies present in the cytoplasm of septic neutrophils. They are approximately 1.3 μm in diameter and consist of endoplasmic reticulum and are present in cases of inflammation/cellulitis and septicaemia.

Leukaemoid reaction

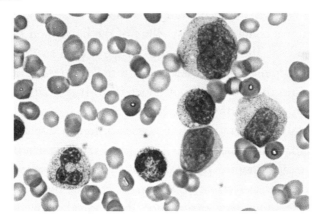

Leukaemoid reaction: Peripheral blood film showing a response to cytokine (G-CSF) therapy (×1000).

A leukaemoid reaction is one in which there is proliferation in the myeloid lineage resulting in a blood picture resembling leukaemia. There is a marked increase in the number of neutrophils together with an increase in the number of myeloblasts, promyelocytes, myelocytes, metamyelocytes and band forms. Leukaemoid reactions may be associated with bacterial reactions, cytokine therapy such as G-CSF and GM-CSF or severe illness such as malignancy. Hypergranulated neutrophils are often a feature of leukaemoid reactions.

Kawasaki disease

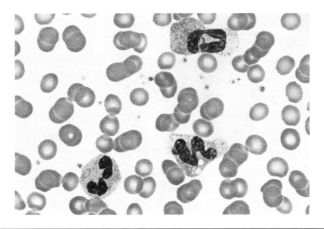

Kawasaki disease: Peripheral blood film from a three-year-old child with a prolonged high fever and rash. The neutrophils show the presence of primary granules, vacuolation and cytoplasmic swelling of the neutrophil membrane (×1000).

A typical blood film in Kawasaki disease shows a normocytic, normochromic anaemia with marked rouleaux formation. The neutrophils show increased granulation and vacuolation. They also show cytoplasmic swelling, a characteristic feature of Kawasaki disease. A marked thrombocytosis is also a feature.

Tomisaku Kawasaki, a Japanese paediatrician, described 50 children with fever lasting for more than five days. The children had cervical lymphadenopathy, rash, bilateral non-exudative conjunctivitis, swelling of the hands and feet and inflammation of the oral mucosa. The children ranged in age from 6 to 12 months. Kawasaki disease is more common amongst males with a male-to-female ratio of 1.5:1. The aetiology of Kawasaki disease is still not understood. It is thought to be a multisystem vasculitic disorder. The onset of the fever is abrupt. It is a high, sustained fever, unresponsive to antibiotic therapy, lasting a week or longer. During the acute phase, Kawasaki disease may cause medium to large vessel arteritis, arterial aneurysms and myocarditis. If untreated, approximately 20% of patients will develop coronary aneurysms. Kawasaki disease has surpassed rheumatic fever as the leading cause of heart disease in children less than five years of age. The medical management of Kawasaki disease involves the use of intravenous gamma globulin, 2 grams per kilo body weight as well as aspirin, which is used as an anti-inflammatory agent.

This figure is from a 12-month-old child with Hb of 90 g/l, WBC of 18.6 × 10^9/L, a platelet count of 720 × 10^9/L and an ESR of 110 mm/hr. *Kawasaki disease is diagnosed from a combination of clinical and haematological features. Bacterial sepsis must always be excluded. Monitor the microbiology results for features of sepsis. Also be aware that the high dose of gamma globulin can give rise to a haemolytic anaemia several days post treatment. Kawasaki disease can lead to coronary artery aneurysms in early childhood if not treated appropriately. Scientists working with paediatric patients should be ever mindful of this potentially fatal disease.*

Alder–Reilly anomaly

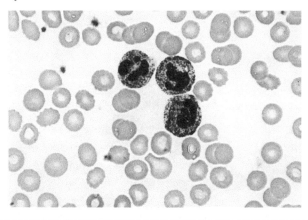

Alder–Reilly anomaly: Peripheral blood film showing neutrophils whose cytoplasm is packed with coarse reddish-brown granules (×1000).

Alder–Reilly anomaly is a mucopolysaccharidosis anomaly where the neutrophils, eosinophils, basophils and monocytes are filled with metachromatic granules of mucopolysaccharide.

When stained with a Romanowsky stain these granules closely resemble granules associated with sepsis. Thus, it is important to distinguish the granules seen in Alder–Reilly anomaly from other disorders associated with hypergranulated neutrophils.

Mucopolysaccharidosis type VI (MPS VI)

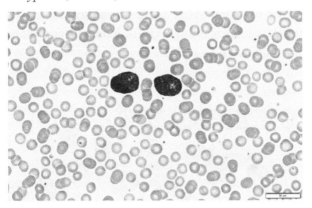

Mucopolysaccharidosis type VI (Maroteaux–Lamy Syndrome) demonstrating neutrophils whose cytoplasm is packed with granules of mucopolysaccharide (×1000).

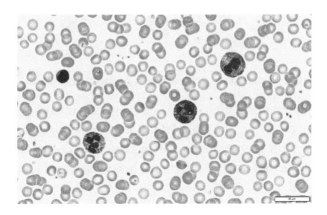

Mucopolysaccharidosis type VI (Maroteaux–Lamy Syndrome) demonstrating neutrophils whose cytoplasm is packed with granules of mucopolysaccharide (×1000).

Also known as Maroteaux–Lamy Syndrome and polydystrophic dwarfism, mucopolysaccharidosis type VI (MPS VI) is inherited as an autosomal recessive trait. Mucopolysaccharidoses are a large group of disorders resulting from a deficiency in one or more lysosomal enzymes. MPS VI is deficient in the lysosomal enzyme known as N-acetylgalactosamine-4-sulfatase. This enzyme breaks down large molecules of sugar known as glycosaminoglycans which are a major constituent of connective tissue. The gene responsible for this enzyme is the arylsulfatase B gene known as the SRSB gene on chromosome 5q14.1.

Lack of this enzyme results in only partially degraded glycosaminoglycan. The accumulated products remaining in the connective tissue, namely dermatan sulphate, lead to clinical features which include severe skeletal dysplasia, short stature, large head and coarse facial features. They develop heart valve abnormalities, breathing difficulties and suffer from sleep apnoea. They develop hearing and vision loss. MPS VI unlike other types of mucopolysaccharidoses does not affect intelligence.

MPS VI is another disorder where the neutrophils closely resemble those seen in Alder–Reilly anomaly and/or sepsis. Again, judicious care should be taken when reporting on hypergranulated neutrophils.

Chédiak–Higashi anomaly

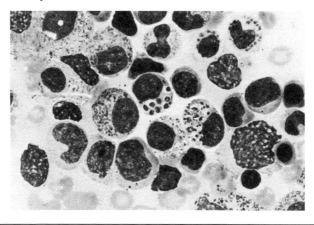

Chédiak–Higashi anomaly: Characteristic giant granules within the cytoplasm of bone marrow myeloid precursors (×1000).

Chédiak–Higashi anomaly is characterised by giant granules in the cytoplasm of neutrophils and lymphocytes. The granules result from the fusion of primary and secondary granules to form giant granules. These giant granules are not attracted to the phagocytic vacuole during bacterial infections; hence bactericidal activity is impaired.

Basophilia/mastocytosis

An absolute basophilia is associated with hypersensitivity reactions to food substances or drugs; it may also occur in conjunction with acute urticaria.

Cutaneous mastocytosis (CM)

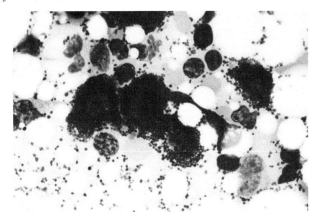

Cutaneous mastocytosis: Bone marrow from an 18-month-old child suffering from an itchy red rash since birth. The bone marrow is heavily infiltrated with mast cells. Some of the squashed mast cells have released histamine granules (×1000).

Cutaneous mastocytosis (CM) occurs in very young children, sometimes presenting at birth. It presents either as a solitary mastocytoma or as uriticaria pigmentosa. Only in rare cases does it involve the bone marrow and progress to mast cell leukaemia. A generalised itching and heparin-like coagulopathy result from the production of histamine by the mast cell granules. Fatal haemorrhage may result from the heparin-like coagulopathy. CM usually regresses spontaneously during early childhood.

Mast cell leukaemia (MCL)

In mast cell leukaemia (MCL) the number of mast cells equals or exceeds 20% of all the nucleated cells within the bone marrow. The marrow shows a diffuse infiltrate of mast cells that are often atypical in appearance with hypogranular cytoplasm and irregularly shaped nuclei. Nucleoli are often prominent. Should the number of mast cells be less than 10% then a diagnosis of 'aleukaemic' MCL is made.

Neonatal neutrophilia

An absolute neutrophilia, present in the first few days of life, is associated with vaginal birth and hence is not present when birth is by caesarean section. The absolute neutrophil count on day 1 ranges from 4.4 to 21.0 × 10^9/L, and by day 7 falls to between 1.5 and 15.3 × 10^9/L. This early physiological neutrophilia is sometimes left-shifted, with an occasional myeloid precursor (e.g., myelocyte, metamyelocyte or band form) present on the peripheral blood film. Neutrophilia persisting beyond the first few days of life may be indicative of a bacterial infection.

Sepsis in the neonate

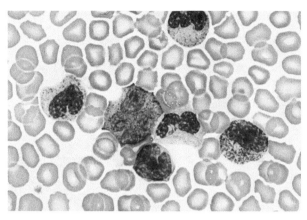

Neonatal sepsis: Hypergranular myeloid precursors in peripheral blood (×1000).

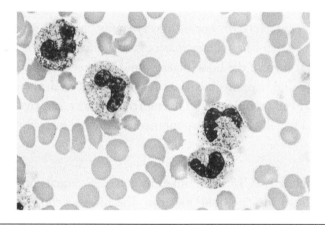

Sepsis at two months of age: Neutrophilia with hypergranular myeloid precursors (×1000).

Diagnosis of neonatal septicaemia is one of the most difficult tasks the neonatologist has to make in clinical medicine. In the neonate bacterial infections have a high mortality rate despite the use of antibiotics. An increase in the number of neutrophils, the presence of hypergranulated neutrophils and a left shift with band forms are all features suggestive of septicaemia. The presence of band forms may be the only indicator of sepsis; hence it is important to count every band form on a neonatal blood film. A ratio of band forms to total neutrophils of 0.2 or higher is suggestive of sepsis.

A band form has no nuclear segmentation. The width of the nucleus at any constriction point is not less than one-third of the width at its widest point. Hypergranulated neutrophils in isolation are not specific for sepsis and may be seen in other conditions such as Alder–Reilly anomaly, Chédiak–Higashi anomaly, cytokine G-CSF therapy and Kawasaki disease.

Bone marrow failure

Aplastic anaemia

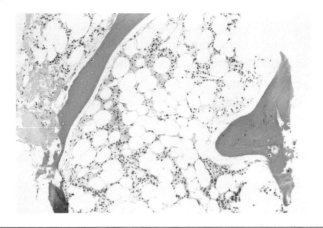

Aplastic anaemia: Hypocellular bone marrow trephine from a two-year-old child showing increased fat spaces (×100).

Aplastic anaemia is a prime example of bone marrow failure. It is characterised by reduced bone marrow production of all three cell lineages: Erythrocytes, granulocytes and platelets. This reduction causes peripheral blood pancytopenia and may be either acquired or inherited. In severe aplastic anaemia, the granulocyte or neutrophil count is <0.5 × 10^9/L, the platelet count is <20 × 10^9/L and the reticulocyte count is <1%. The anaemia may be normocytic or macrocytic. The bone marrow is hypocellular, with empty fragments and increased fat spaces. Aplastic anaemia may be inherited or acquired. Acquired aplastic anaemia may be secondary to certain drugs, chemicals and viruses (parvovirus, Epstein–Barr virus, cytomegalovirus and human immunodeficiency virus). Inherited aplastic anaemia includes disorders such as Fanconi anaemia, dyskeratosis congenita and Shwachman–Diamond syndrome.

Dyskeratosis congenita (DC)

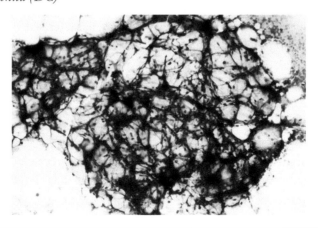

Dyskeratosis congenita: Hypocellular bone marrow fragment in a 12-year-old child (×100).

Dyskeratosis congenita (DC) is a disorder of the mucocutaneous and haemopoietic systems. The mucocutaneous aspect of the disorder is characterised by a triad of events: Pigmentation of the upper body, mucosal leucoplakia and nail dystrophy. The haemopoietic aspect of the disorder is characterised by aplastic anaemia occurring in the second decade of life and in approximately 50% of cases. A small percentage of cases have a predisposition to develop cancer in the third to fourth decade of life. DC has three patterns of inheritance: X-linked recessive, autosomal recessive and autosomal-dominant. The haematological features of DC are anaemia, leucopoenia and thrombocytopenia. The bone marrow is initially hypercellular but gradually becomes hypocellular, culminating in aplastic anaemia. The red cells are macrocytic and HbF is increased. Chromosome fragility in DC is variable when diepoxybutane (DEB) is added to culture.

Pancytopenias

Fanconi anaemia (FA)
Fanconi anaemia (FA) is an autosomal-recessive disorder encompassing a group of patients with familial aplastic anaemia and physical anomalies. There is clinical variability amongst patients with FA. Three groups of patients have been described: Those with physical anomalies and normal haematological findings, those with no physical anomaly but with abnormal haematological findings and those with both a physical anomaly and abnormal haematological findings. The haematological features in Fanconi anaemia lead to the gradual onset of bone marrow failure. Patients present initially with thrombocytopenia that is followed by neutropenia and then anaemia. The red cells are often macrocytic with a mean cell volume (MCV) of more than 100 fL. There is an increase in HbF production. Erythropoietin levels are also increased. The bone marrow is hypercellular in early FA (before the development of pancytopenia). When the patient becomes aplastic, the bone marrow is hypocellular and fatty with few haematopoietic elements. There is an increase in the number of lymphocytes, reticulum cells, mast cells and plasma cells. FA is characterised by abnormal chromosome fragility. Spontaneous breaks, gaps, rearrangements and endoreduplications occur. This abnormal chromosome fragility can be exacerbated by the addition of DEB in chromosome culture. FA homozygotes have a mean of 8.96 breaks per cell with DEB culture compared with 0.06 breaks in normal subjects.

Shwachman–Diamond syndrome (SDS)
Shwachman–Diamond syndrome (SDS) is an autosomal-recessive disorder characterised by pancreatic dysfunction, malabsorption, steatorrhea, failure to thrive, short stature and (in some cases) mental retardation. Fatty infiltration of the pancreas leads to pancreatic insufficiency with low or absent duodenal trypsin, amylase and lipase. The main haematological feature of SDS is neutropenia. Anaemia and thrombocytopenia may occur in some cases. The neutropenia is intermittent rather than constant

and is associated with skin infections and pneumonia. Abnormal neutrophil mobility, migration and chemotaxis lead to recurrent infections. An increase in HbF, even without anaemia is common. Bone marrow hypoplasia with maturation arrest in the myeloid line is present. Chromosomes are normal and there is no increased breakage following clastogenic stress with DEB.

Neutropenia

Cyclic neutropenia

Cyclic neutropenia is a rare disorder characterised by severe neutropenia lasting 3–6 days in a 21-day cycle. During this neutropenic phase, the absolute neutrophil count is <0.2 × 10⁹/L and the bone marrow shows a maturation arrest at the myelocyte stage. Monocytes, lymphocytes, eosinophils, platelets and reticulocytes also demonstrate cycling. The majority of patients experience oral ulcers, stomatitis and pharyngitis with lymphadenopathy during the neutropenic stage. The severity of the infection parallels the degree of neutropenia. G-CSF is widely used in cyclic neutropenia. It increases the neutrophil count, thus preventing transient infections during the neutropenic phase. Evidence for genetic transmission has been noted in about 25% of families with cyclic neutropenia. The mode of inheritance is autosomal-recessive. However, in other cases, the disease occurs spontaneously.

Kostmann syndrome

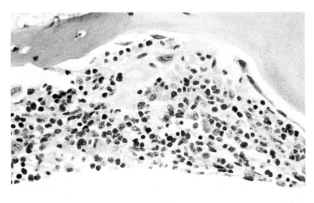

Kostmann syndrome: Bone marrow trephine showing marked neutropenia (H&E) (×400).

Kostmann syndrome is a severe congenital neutropenia occurring in early childhood. The mode of inheritance of Kostmann syndrome is autosomal-recessive. Absolute neutrophil counts of <0.2 × 10⁹/L are characteristic, while the bone marrow shows a maturation arrest at the promyelocyte/myelocyte stage. A compensatory monocytosis as well as eosinophilia may be present. Some children with Kostmann syndrome develop bacterial infections in the first few weeks of life and almost all cases develop infections by the age of six months. Skin abscesses, fungal infections and septicaemia are commonly seen. Kostmann syndrome is responsive to cytokines. G-CSF raises the neutrophil count to such a level that infection and septicaemia are rarely seen. This results in a dramatic improvement in the quality of life for children with Kostmann syndrome.

Eosinophilia

Eosinophilia in the neonate

Eosinophils can occur in the neonatal period. The duration of the eosinophilia can be in excess of six weeks, especially in those infants with a high absolute eosinophil count. The majority of neonatal cases of eosinophilia are associated with gram-negative infections such as necrotising enterocolitis (NEC).

Eosinophilia in early childhood

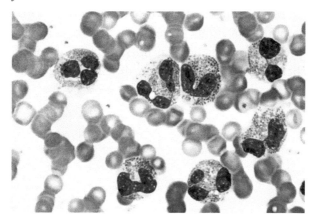

Eosinophilia: Parasitic infection: Peripheral blood film from a child infected with *Toxocara canis* showing a marked eosinophilia. The absolute eosinophil count on this child was 46.4 × 10⁹/L (×1000).

Eosinophilia occurs in allergic reactions such as hay fever, asthma and milk-protein colitis. The intake of cow's milk may lead to allergic eosinophilia. Eosinophilia also occurs in parasitic infections of the gastrointestinal tract. *Toxocara canis* infection may result in a marked systemic reaction with persistent eosinophilia lasting many years. No causative agent has been found in a significant number of cases of eosinophilia. Many of these cases resolve slowly over a period of time.

Leucoerythroblastosis

Osteopetrosis

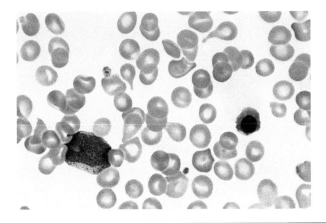

Osteopetrosis: Peripheral blood film showing leucoerythroblastic blood picture with teardrop poikilocytes from a seven-week-old infant with the malignant form of osteopetrosis (×1000).

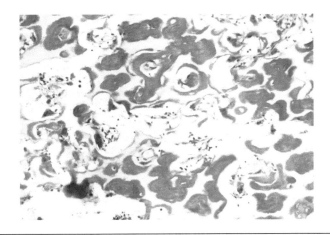

Osteopetrosis: Bone marrow trephine showing the 'marble bone' effect in a young child (H&E) (×50).

Osteopetrosis or Albers–Schönberg disease is often referred to as 'marble bone' disease. The osteoclasts in osteopetrosis, although normal in number and morphology, are functionally abnormal in that they are unable to reabsorb and remodel bone. This defect results in loss of haemopoietic tissue due to obliteration of the marrow cavity. Two forms of osteopetrosis occur depending on the mode of inheritance. The milder form is inherited as an autosomal-dominant disorder. It is diagnosed in late childhood and is characterised by the presence of sclerotic bones that fracture easily. There are no specific haematological findings associated with the milder form.

The severe or malignant form of osteopetrosis is inherited as an autosomal-recessive disorder. It is diagnosed in infancy or early childhood and is also characterised by the presence of dense sclerotic bones. This more severe form is associated with clinical abnormalities such as microcephaly, blindness, deafness and cranial nerve palsies.

Haematological complications are severe in the malignant form of osteopetrosis. They include anaemia, leucopenia and thrombocytopenia. The red cells are macrocytic. The blood film is leucoerythroblastic, with teardrop poikilocytes.

Myeloproliferative neoplasms in the neonate and childhood

Transient abnormal myelopoiesis (TAM)

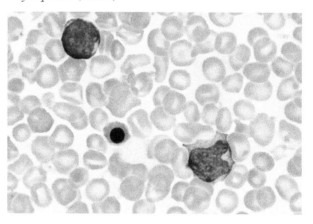

Transient abnormal myelopoiesis. Peripheral blood film from a newborn with Down syndrome. Two blast cells (megakaryo-blasts) and a NRBC are present. The white cell count is 15.8 × 10⁹/L and the absolute blast cell count is 5.2 × 10⁹/L (×1000).

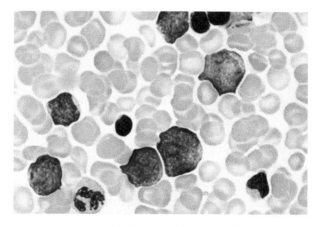

Transient abnormal myelopoiesis: Bone marrow from the above case showing a proliferation of blast cells. The blast cells are pleomorphic with some cytoplasmic budding, suggestive of megakaryoblastic leukaemia (×1000).

Transient abnormal myelopoiesis (TAM) may occur in the neonatal period. It is often associated with Down syndrome (trisomy 21) and morphologically closely resembles acute myeloid leukaemia (AML). TAM is characterised by an uncontrolled proliferation of blasts that regress spontaneously within weeks or months. This myeloproliferative disorder is associated with a hepatosplenomegaly. The haemoglobin is usually normal while the platelet count is reduced with large and giant platelets present.

TAM may be confused with congenital leukaemia in the initial stages or until spontaneous remission occurs within the first three months of life. Twenty-five percent of cases of TAM will go on to develop acute megakaryoblastic leukaemia by the age of three years. In approximately 20–30% of cases with Down syndrome, the blast cells will persist and a true congenital leukaemia will develop. Acute lymphoblastic as well as acute myeloblastic leukaemia may occur in children with Down syndrome. The most frequently occurring myeloblastic leukaemia is megakaryoblastic leukaemia.

Cytogenetics: In addition to the trisomy 21 of Down syndrome, no specific chromosomal abnormalities are associated with transient abnormal myelopoiesis.

Immunophenotype: The markers expressed by TAM resemble those expressed by megakaryoblastic leukaemia: HLA-DR$^{-/+}$, CD34$^+$, CD56$^+$, CD117$^+$, CD13$^+$, CD33$^+$, CD7$^+$, CD45$^-$, CD41$^+$, CD61$^+$.

Monocytes and macrophages

Monocytic maturation

Monocytes are produced in the bone marrow. They migrate to the peripheral blood and then to organs of the reticuloendothelial system. Monocytes differentiate into macrophages or histiocytes. They then migrate to the tissues where they act as phagocytes. In the tissues, they clear the body of microbial organisms and of age-damaged cells by a process of pinocytosis and phagocytosis.

The maturation of monocytes is divided into three stages: The monoblast, promonocyte and mature monocyte.

Monoblast

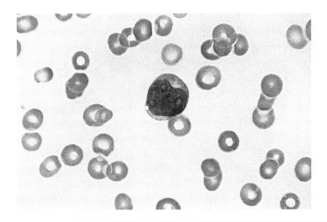

Monoblast (×1000).

The monoblast varies in diameter from 14 to 18 μm. It has a round to oval nucleus occupying about 80% of the cell and one or two nucleoli. The cytoplasm is basophilic and lacks granules.

Promonocyte

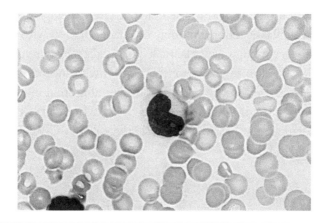

Promonocyte (×1000).

The promonocyte varies in diameter from 14 to 18 μm. The nucleus is indented and often contains a nucleolus. The cytoplasm is blue-grey and may contain a few fine azurophilic granules.

Monocyte

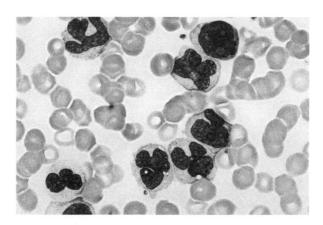

Monocytes and a single monoblast (×1000).

The monocyte varies from 12 to 18 μm. The nucleus is folded and lobulated with two or more lobes. The cytoplasm is grey-blue with numerous fine azurophilic granules. Vacuolation is a characteristic feature of the mature monocyte.

Disorders of the monocyte/macrophage system involve monocytic proliferation in the blood and bone marrow as well as congenital and acquired macrophage disorders. Monocyte proliferative disorders are closely associated with the myeloid line of cells involving leukaemic states, for example, myelodysplastic syndrome, juvenile myelomonocytic leukaemia and myelomonocytic leukaemia. A small number of cases of chronic monocytic leukaemia have also been described.

Gaucher disease

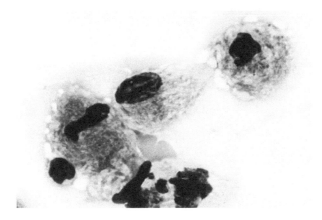

Gaucher disease: Bone marrow showing Gaucher macrophages with a striated pattern within the cytoplasm that resembles the skin of an onion (×1000).

Gaucher disease is a lipid storage disease characterised by the presence of macrophages throughout the bone marrow and organs of the reticuloendothelial system. These macrophages known as Gaucher cells measure between 20 and 100 μm in diameter and have a striated cytoplasm resembling onion skin that is due to the accumulation of glucocerebroside stored within their cytoplasm. The fundamental biochemical defect is due to a severe reduction of the enzyme glucocerebroside β-glucosidase, which catalyses the hydrolytic splitting-off of glucose in normal tissues, including peripheral leucocytes. Gaucher disease is recessively inherited and is found in all populations but has a higher frequency amongst Ashkenazi Jews. The principal features of the disease include a massive splenomegaly and, less frequently, hepatomegaly. Anaemia and thrombocytopenia are usually present, leading to the need for a splenectomy in such patients. Laboratory diagnosis depends upon the presence of Gaucher cells in the bone marrow as well as the demonstration of deficiency in lysosomal β-glucosidase activity measured in leucocytes.

Niemann–Pick disease

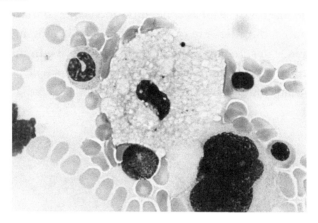

Niemann–Pick disease: Bone marrow showing a foamy macrophage whose cytoplasm is filled with droplets of ceroid (×1000).

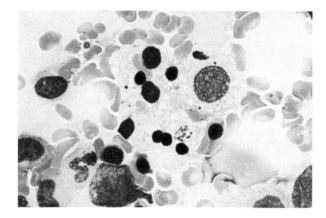

Niemann–Pick disease: Bone marrow showing a foamy macrophage that has phagocytosed several lymphocyte nuclei (×1000).

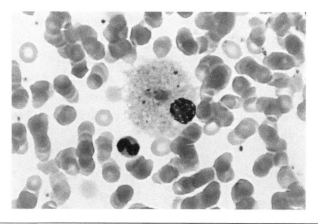

Niemann–Pick disease: Bone marrow showing a sea-blue histiocyte filled with large blue granules containing ceroid (×1000).

Niemann–Pick disease is characterised by a deficiency of the enzyme sphingomy-elinase leading to a build-up of sphingomyelin, cholesterol and other cell membrane lipids which accumulate within foam cells throughout the reticuloendothelial system. Foam cells range in size from 20 to 10 μm in diameter and their cytoplasm is packed with small droplets of lipid – hence the description of 'foam' cells. The presence of these cells in the bone marrow provides the simplest means for diagnosis. Sea-blue histiocytes are also present in the bone marrow of Niemann–Pick disease. The cyto-plasm of these histiocytes is filled with large granules containing ceroid that stain greenish-blue with Romanowsky stains. Niemann–Pick disease is recessively inher-ited and is also found in high frequency among Ashkenazi Jews. Anaemia may be present in some patients but the majority of cases have a normal haemoglobin level. On examination of the blood film, the majority of lymphocytes is noted to contain cytoplasmic vacuolation. The vacuoles represent lipid-filled lysosomes.

Reactive haemophagocytic syndrome

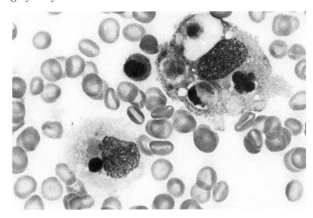

Reactive haemophagocytosis syndrome: Macrophages present in the bone marrow of a six-year-old child that have phago-cytosed red cells and white cell nuclei (×1000).

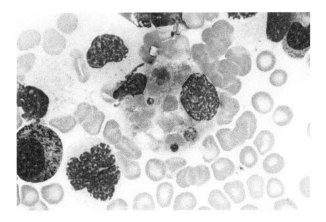

Reactive haemophagocytosis syndrome: Bone marrow from the case above showing a macrophage that has phagocytosed erythrocytes (×1000).

This is characterised by a proliferation of macrophages or histiocytes within organs of the reticuloendothelial system. The syndrome may be associated with a systemic viral infection such as Epstein–Barr virus (EBV), cytomegalovirus (CMV), herpes simplex or varicella. Sometimes the syndrome may be associated with a bacterial, fungal or protozoal infection. It may also occur in malignant histiocytosis. The clinical signs of the syndrome include fever, lethargy and myalgia. Young children often have an associated splenomegaly or hepatosplenomegaly. The clinical signs of the syndrome include fever, lethargy and myalgia. Young children often have an associated splenomegaly or hepatosplenomegaly. Patients present with severe anaemia, leucopoenia and thrombocytopenia. Bone marrow examination reveals an increase in macrophages, many of which have phagocytosed erythrocytes, leucocytes and platelets.

Langerhans cell histiocytosis (LCH)

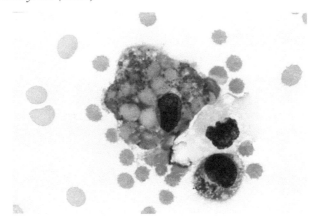

Langerhans cell histiocytosis (histiocytosis X) fine-needle biopsy of the parotid gland of a three-year-old child showing histiocytic erythrophagocytosis (×1000).

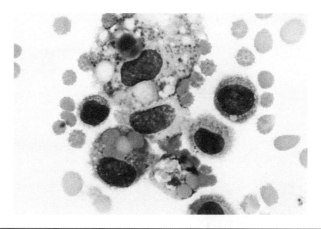

Langerhans cell histiocytosis (histiocytosis X) fine-needle biopsy of the parotid gland of a three-year-old child showing a histiocyte which has phagocytosed red cells, white cell nuclei and platelets (×1000).

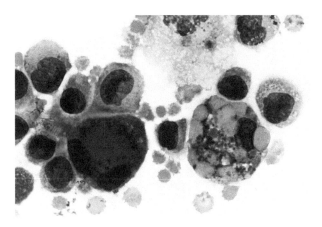

Langerhans cell histiocytosis (histiocytosis X) fine-needle biopsy of the parotid gland of a three-year-old child showing histiocytic erythrophagocytosis (×1000).

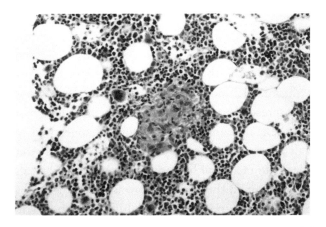

Bone marrow trephine from a child with sarcoidosis showing a large granuloma (H&E) (×400).

Langerhans cell histiocytosis (LCH) (histiocytosis X) affects mainly children in the first four years of life but may occur in patients 20 years and under. It is categorised according to the level of dissemination. It can be localised, infiltrating the skin, skull, ribs and long bones. It can also be disseminated, involving the lymph nodes, liver, spleen and bone marrow. In disseminated LCH the bone marrow contains lipid-laden macrophages and eosinophilic granulomas. Localised disease in bone is associated with a peripheral blood eosinophilia.

Storage disorders in the neonate and childhood

α-*mannosidosis*

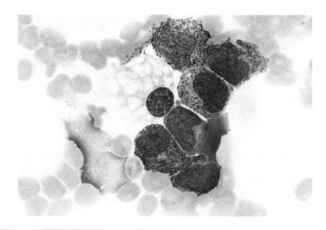

α-mannosidosis: Bone marrow showing the presence of a foamy macrophage (×1000).

α-mannosidosis is an oligosaccharide storage disease characterised by deficiency of the enzyme α-mannosidase. There are two phenotypes: The infantile phenotype, which presents in the first 12 months of life and has a short survival and the juvenile/adult phenotype, presenting later in life and having a longer survival. The clinical features include skeletal changes, coarse facial changes and mental retardation. Hepatosplenomegaly is present in the early stage of the disease. Abnormal chemotaxis of the neutrophils leads to recurrent bacterial infections. The circulating lymphocytes have vacuolated cytoplasm and the bone marrow is packed with foamy macrophages. The lymphocyte vacuoles show periodic acid Schiff (PAS) positivity. Increased levels of mannosidase-containing oligosaccharides are found in the tissues as well as in the urine.

Mucopolysaccharidoses
Mucopolysaccharidosis storage disorders lead to morphological changes in white cells in both the peripheral blood and the bone marrow. Mucopolysaccharides are complex carbohydrates found in various types of connective tissue, including cartilage and bone. The presence of excessive amounts of mucopolysaccharide leads to coarse facial features, skeletal dysplasia and limitation of joint movement (Hurler syndrome). Mucopolysaccharidosis results from a lysosomal enzyme deficiency.

Hurler syndrome (Gasser lymphocytes)

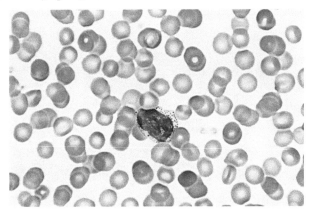

Hurler syndrome: Peripheral blood film from a child with Hurler syndrome showing a classical Gasser lymphocyte whose cytoplasm is filled with clear vacuoles containing large coarse metachromatic granules of mucopolysaccharide (×1000).

Hurler syndrome, a mucopolysaccharide storage disorder, is characterised by the presence of lymphocytes whose cytoplasm contains clear vacuoles filled with coarse metachromatic granules of mucopolysaccharide. These lymphocytes have been described by Gasser and are known as Gasser lymphocytes.

Cystinosis

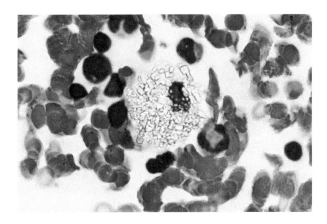

Cystinosis: Bone marrow showing the presence of a macrophage whose cytoplasm is packed with rectangular shaped crystals of cysteine (×1000).

Cystinosis is an autosomal-recessive disorder that first presents at 6–12 months of age. The clinical characteristics of this disorder include failure to thrive, progressive renal failure, loss of muscle function, photophobia and fair hair. The bone marrow is characterised by the presence of macrophages packed with rectangular-shaped crystals of cysteine. Rarely can these be seen in the peripheral blood. Diagnosis of cystinosis is by way of a biochemical assay rather than by bone marrow examination. The cysteine content of the white cells is measured. This is because the aqueous staining solutions used to stain the crystals tend to dissolve much of the cysteine, leaving few crystals visible under the light microscope.

Wolman disease

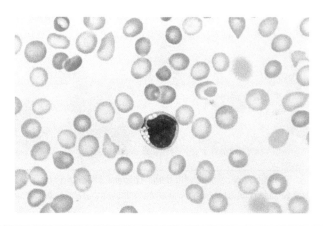

Wolman disease: Peripheral blood film from a four-week-neonate showing characteristic vacuolation in the cytoplasm of a lymphocyte (×1000).

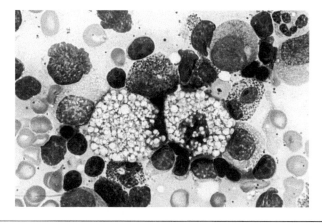

Wolman disease: Foamy macrophages present in the bone marrow of the above neonate (×1000).

Wolman disease is an autosomal-recessive disorder. It is characterised by an abnormality in the lysosomal acid lipase (LIPA) gene resulting in a deficiency of the acid cholesteryl ester hydrolase enzyme. Deficiency of this enzyme leads to an accumulation of cholesterol and triglycerides within the body organs and tissues. The clinical features of Wolman disease include steatorrhea, hepatosplenomegaly, intestinal malabsorption, abdominal protuberance, poor weight gain and diffuse punctate adrenal calcification. Xanthomatous changes are seen in the liver, the adrenal glands, the spleen, the lymph nodes, the small intestine, the lungs and the thymus and, to a lesser extent, the skin. The peripheral blood is characterised by the presence of vacuolated lymphocytes and the bone marrow by the presence of foamy macrophages. The vacuoles in both the lymphocytes and bone marrow macrophages stain positively with oil red O stain and Sudan black B stain. Normal to moderately elevated levels of plasma lipids and hypercholesterolaemia are present. Death occurs in early infancy.

Monosomy 7 myeloproliferative disease (MPD)

Monosomy 7 myeloproliferative disease (MPD) has been referred to as a 'subleukaemic' disorder occurring in young children, usually less than five years of age. It affects boys more frequently than girls. These children have a long history of recurrent infections and abnormal neutrophil function. They have a leucocytosis with a left shift in the myeloid lineage as well as an absolute monocytosis, anaemia and thrombocytopenia. The bone marrow is hypercellular and often dysplastic. HbF is either normal or slightly raised. Monosomy 7 often progresses to acute myeloblastic leukaemia.

Cytogenetics-7/del(7q)

Juvenile myelomonocytic leukaemia (JMML)

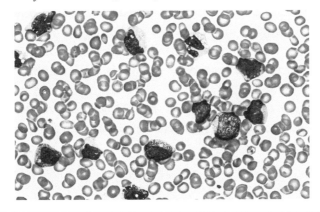

Juvenile myelomonocytic leukaemia: Peripheral blood film from a four-year-old child (×1000).

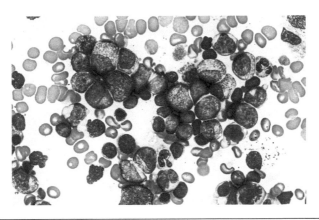

Juvenile myelomonocytic leukaemia: Bone marrow from the above patient showing myeloid precursors, blasts and occasional NRBC (×1000).

Juvenile myelomonocytic leukaemia (JMML) is a clonal neoplasm characterised by an increase in granulocytes and monocytes. It occurs mainly in children from one month to 14 years of age with the majority of cases occurring in children less than three years of age. The neoplasm is more common in males than females. It is sometimes preceded by an eczematous rash that when biopsied shows a leukaemic infiltrate. Ten percent of cases are associated with the clinical disorder neurofibromatosis type 1. JMML is characterised by an elevated white cell count that is usually <100 × 10^9/L with <20% blasts (plus promonocytes) in the peripheral blood and bone marrow. Dysplasia in JMML is mild, occurring more often in the granulocyte lineage than in the erythroid or megakaryocytic lineage. Haemoglobin F is increased for age. It ranges from 38 to 70% of total haemoglobin with a uniform distribution throughout the red cells. HbA_2 is normal or decreased.

Cytogenetics: The *BCR-ABL1* fusion gene and Ph chromosome are absent. Monosomy 7 occurs in approximately 25% of cases but is not specific for JMML.

Myelodysplastic syndromes (MDS)

Myelodysplastic syndromes (MDS) are rarely seen in childhood. They are usually associated with other conditions such as Down syndrome, Fanconi anaemia, Kostmann syndrome, Diamond–Blackfan anaemia and Schwachman–Diamond syndrome.

MDS may also occur as de novo or be secondary to chemotherapy given for some other malignancy.

When commenting on the blood film from a patient who is being treated with Methotrexate for example for a known malignancy, review the clinical notes before reporting features of MDS on the blood film.

Lymphocytes

Lymphocyte maturation

Lymphocytes develop mainly in the lymphoid tissues of the body, namely the lymph nodes, the spleen and the lymphoid follicles within the bone marrow. Lymphatic maturation is divided into three stages: The lymphoblast, prolymphocyte and lymphocyte (large and small). Maturation proceeds along two pathways: One in the thymus producing T lymphocytes (CD4 and CD8 cells) and the other in lymph nodes producing B lymphocytes.

Lymphoblast

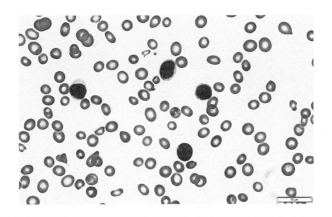

Lymphoblasts in peripheral blood (×1000).

The lymphoblast varies from 10 to 20 μm in diameter. It has a round nucleus that occupies about 80% of the cell. The chromatin is fine and contains one to two nucleoli. The cytoplasm is basophilic and agranular.

Prolymphocyte

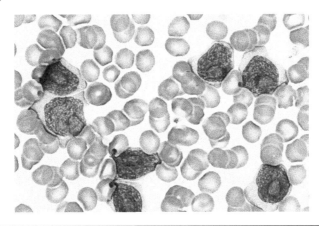

Prolymphocytes in peripheral blood (×1000).

The prolymphocyte varies in diameter from 10 to 18 μm. The nucleus is round, the chromatin denser and the cytoplasm more abundant compared with the lymphoblast. One prominent nucleolus is present within the nucleus.

Lymphocyte (small)

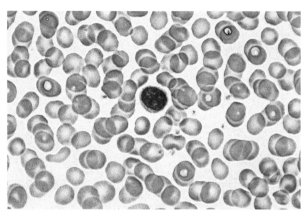

Small lymphocyte in peripheral blood (×1000).

The small lymphocyte varies in diameter from 9 to 12 μm. The nucleus is round, with coarse clumped chromatin. The cytoplasm is scanty, sky blue in colour and agranular. It may be a T or B lymphocyte; differentiation between the two can only be achieved by examining immune surface markers.

Lymphocyte (large)

The large lymphocyte varies in diameter from 12 to 16 μm. The nucleus is round, with coarse clumped chromatin. The cytoplasm is abundant and sky blue in colour and often contains a few azurophilic granules. Large granular lymphocytes are usually $CD8^+$ T lymphocytes.

Reactive lymphocytosis

Reactive lymphocytosis occurs in a number of viral illnesses: Infectious mononucleosis, cytomegalovirus infection and viral hepatitis. Reactive lymphocytes are also seen in the bacterial infection *Bordetella pertussis* and also in what is described as 'non-specific' acute infectious lymphocytosis. Such reactions must be clearly distinguished from lymphocytic leukaemias.

> *Care must be taken <u>not</u> to describe 'reactive' lymphocytes as 'atypical lymphocytes.' A reactive lymphocyte is a $CD8^+T$ cell which is reacting to a pathogen. It is not uncommon to see an occasional reactive lymphocyte in the blood film of young children.*

Reactive lymphocytes (infectious mononucleosis) (IM)

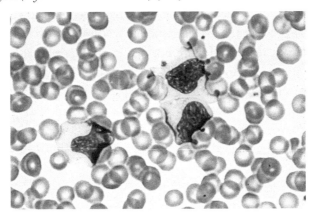

Reactive lymphocytes in a case of infectious mononucleosis showing basophilic flowing cytoplasm with dark-staining periphery (×1000).

Infectious mononucleosis (IM) is an infection caused by the Epstein–Barr virus (EBV) and occurs in teenagers and young adults. The clinical presentation includes lassitude, fever, pharyngitis, lymphadenopathy and hepatosplenomegaly. The blood film shows a proliferation of virally infected B lymphocytes with about 20% or more reactive lymphocytes that are activated T lymphocytes. These reactive lymphocytes have round or irregularly shaped nuclei, with abundant flowing cytoplasm that characteristically has a dark-staining periphery. Thrombocytopenia is a common feature in EBV infection. IM is heterophile antibody positive, thus distinguishing it from other virally induced lymphoproliferative disorders, which are all heterophile antibody negative. Some patients also present with a haemolytic anaemia resulting from the production of antibodies by the B lymphocytes against the 'I' antigen on the red cells. In such cases, a degree of auto-agglutination of the red cells is seen on the blood film.

Cytomegalovirus (CMV) infection

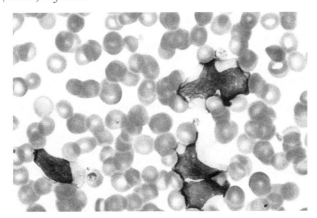

Cytomegalovirus infection: Peripheral blood film showing reactive T lymphocytes morphologically indistinguishable from those of an Epstein–Barr virus infection showing irregularly shaped nuclei and flowing basophilic cytoplasm with dark-staining periphery (×1000).

Cytomegalovirus (CMV) infection usually occurs in patients between the ages of 20 and 50 years. The virus infects the neutrophils which spread the infection to the macrophages. This produces a T-cell response leading to a lymphocytosis and the presence of circulating reactive T lymphocytes in the peripheral blood. The clinical features of CMV are similar to those of IM with two exceptions: Patients with CMV rarely present with pharyngitis or lymphadenopathy. The lymphocytes of CMV are morphologically indistinguishable from those of an EBV infection; the main difference between the two illnesses is that the CMV infection is heterophile antibody negative. Thrombocytopenia is also a common feature of CMV infection.

Varicella infection

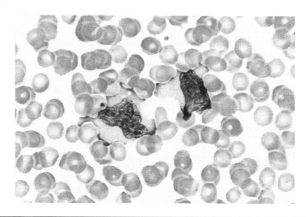

Varicella infection: Peripheral blood film showing reactive T lymphocytes with irregularly shaped nuclei and basophilic flowing cytoplasm (×1000).

Varicella infection (chicken pox) is commonly seen in young children but may also occur in adulthood. The classical features are thrombocytopenia and the presence in the peripheral blood of reactive T lymphocytes closely resembling those induced by EBV and CMV infections.

Viral hepatitis

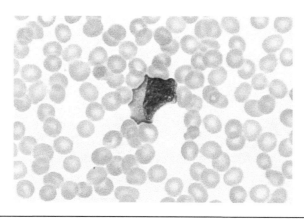

Viral hepatitis: Peripheral blood film showing a reactive lymphocyte with similar characteristics to those found in other viral infections (×1000).

Both hepatitis A and B viruses can produce a mononucleosis-like syndrome characterised by reactive lymphocytes on the blood film.

Bordetella pertussis

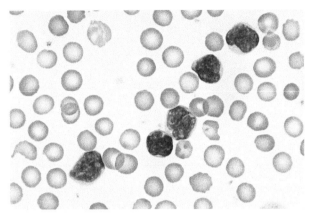

Bordetella pertussis: Peripheral blood film showing T lymphocytes with cleaved nuclei (×1000).

Bordetella pertussis is a gram-negative coccobacillus that is the cause of a highly contagious disease known as 'whooping cough.' *Bordetella pertussis* infects its host by colonising the epithelial cells in the lung. The bacteria have a surface protein known as 'filamentous haemagglutinin adhesion' which binds to the sulfatides on the cilia of the epithelial cells lining the nose and throat. Once anchored on the cilia, the bacteria produce a tracheal toxin known as *pertussis* toxin which paralyses the cilia, preventing them from beating. This leads to inflammation of the respiratory tract, interfering with the clearance of pulmonary secretions and debris from the lungs. The body responds by sending the host into a coughing fit which expels bacteria into the air, free to infect other hosts. The characteristic 'whoop' is made as the infected host struggles to breathe through narrowed airway passages between coughing spasms.

The *Pertussis* toxin, referred to as a lymphocytosis-promoting factor, causes a decrease in the entry of lymphocytes into the lymph nodes thus there is a build-up of lymphocytes in the peripheral blood. A morphological feature of these T cells is that they often have a cleaved nucleus.

Acute infectious lymphocytosis

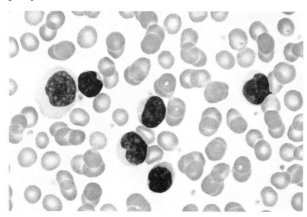

Acute infectious lymphocytosis: Morphologically normal T lymphocytes present in the peripheral blood film from a three-year-old child with an absolute lymphocyte count of 39 × 10⁹/L (×1000).

Acute infectious lymphocytosis occurs in children between the ages of 1 and 14 years, with the highest incidence in the first ten years of life. It may be associated with a low-grade fever and diarrhoea. The absolute lymphocyte count is very high. It can reach $50 \times 10^9/L$ and the majority of lymphocytes are CD4⁺ T lymphocytes. The condition resolves in 2–4 weeks without treatment. Acute infectious lymphocytosis is thought to be associated with a viral infection.

Sialic acid storage disease

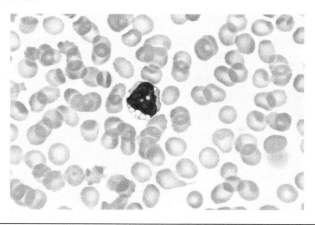

Sialic acid storage disease: Peripheral blood film from a two-month-old child showing a characteristic vacuolated lymphocyte (×1000).

Sialic acid storage disease is a rare inherited autosomal-recessive disorder resulting from a block in sialic acid release from cell lysosomes. The accumulation of sialic acid in many cells, including lymphocytes, leads to cytoplasmic vacuolation. Sialic storage disease is diagnosed by the presence of increased amounts sialic acid in blood, urine and lymphocytes. The disease presents in two forms: A severe form occurring in early life, named infantile sialic acid storage disease (ISSD) and a less aggressive form, named Salla disease after the region in Finland where it was first recognised. The infantile form is characterised by coarse facial features, lack of skin pigmentation, hepatosplenomegaly and anaemia progressing to fluid retention, ascites, heart failure and early death. Salla disease has similar features as well as mental retardation and cerebella ataxia.

Non-haemopoietic malignancies in the neonate and childhood

Neuroblastoma

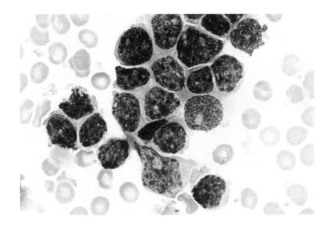

Neuroblastoma: A clump of tumour cells in the marrow characterised by a relatively high N/C ratio and a tendency to form clumps (×1000).

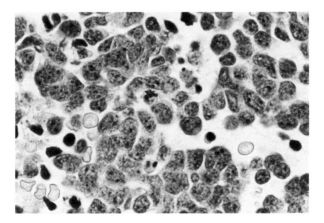

Neuroblastoma: Bone marrow trephine showing sheets of neuroblastoma cells with prominent nuclei (H&E) (×1000).

Neuroblastoma is a tumour of developing sympathetic nervous tissue. It is an embryonal tumour and usually presents in the first five years of life. It occurs in any site where sympathetic nerve tissue is found, namely the adrenal medulla and the paraspinal sympathetic ganglia. In about 50% of cases, neuroblastoma is found infiltrating the bone marrow. Neuroblastoma cells have a tendency to form clumps and rosettes on bone marrow films. The process of aspirating the bone marrow may result in physical disruption of these clumps leaving bare nuclei and cytoplasmic or stromal debris over the marrow film. Neuroblastoma is associated with a normocytic normochromic anaemia, but in cases where there has been bleeding into the tumour, the red cells may be microcytic and hypochromic. The platelet count is usually increased, as is the ESR (>50 mm/h). Tumour cells are rarely seen on the peripheral blood film.

Rhabdomyosarcoma

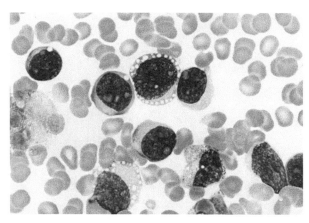

Rhabdomyosarcoma: Bone marrow showing individual tumour cells with prominent vacuolation (×1000).

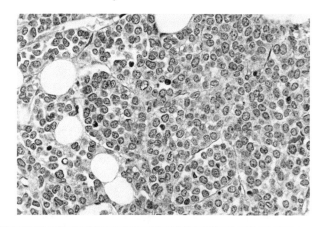

Rhabdomyosarcoma: Bone marrow trephine showing infiltrate of rhabdomyosarcoma cells (H&E) (×1000).

Rhabdomyosarcoma is the most common soft tissue malignancy occurring in children. It is a tumour of striated muscle and only involves the bone marrow in 25–30% of cases. Rhabdomyosarcoma cells in the marrow appear as large cells with prominent vacuolation. The vacuoles often coalesce into elongated lakes and stain positively with PAS reagent. Rhabdomyosarcoma may arise anywhere in the body: The head, the neck, the retroperitoneum, the genitourinary tract and the extremities. It has two age peaks, the first being between the ages of two and six years and the second between 14 and 18 years.

Ewing sarcoma (EWS)

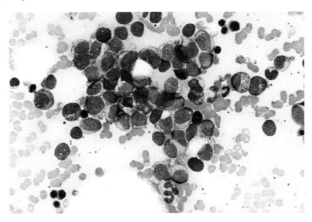

Ewing sarcoma: Bone marrow showing sheets of Ewing sarcoma cells (×400).

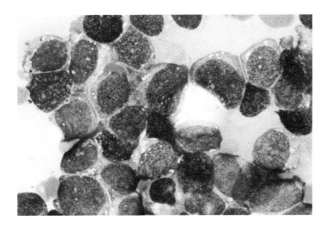

Ewing sarcoma: Bone marrow showing sheets of sarcoma cells with characteristic vacuolated cytoplasm (×1000).

Ewing sarcoma (EWS) is a tumour of bone seen predominantly in the young (less than 20 years of age). It occurs in the femur, the ribs and also the vertebrae and pelvic bones. Ewing sarcoma cells are small, round and undifferentiated. Ewing sarcoma stains positively with PAS reagent

Platelet reference ranges in infancy and childhood

AGE	PLT(x 10^9/L)		PDW(fL)		MPV(fL)	
0-1 d	195	434	9.5	14.5	8.9	11.8
1-7 d	200	500	9.4	14.5	8.7	11.8
1-2 w	250	600	9.4	14.5	8.7	11.8
2w – 3m	270	645	9.4	14.0	8.7	11.0
3-6 m	296	686	8.5	12.3	8.1	10.5
6m – 2y	205	553	8.4	13.1	7.9	10.8
2-4 y	214	483	8.4	13.1	8.0	10.9
4-8 y	205	457	9.0	14.2	8.4	11.5
8-12 y	187	415	9.5	14.2	8.6	11.5

This figure demonstrates the platelet count, the platelet distribution width and the mean platelet volume from 0–1 day to 12 years of age. Note the platelet count is significantly higher than that occurring in normal healthy adults.

This chart demonstrates the platelet count $\times 10^9$/L, the platelet distribution width (PDW) and the mean platelet volume (MPV) ranging from 0–1 day and 12 years of age. Note the platelet count reaches a peak at 3–6 months of age with a count of 686 $\times 10^9$/L.

Megakaryocytic maturation

Megakaryocytic maturation occurs within the bone marrow by a process known as endomytosis. The nucleus replicates in multiples of two without cytoplasmic division, only enlargement of volume. The cytoplasm becomes less basophilic as the mega-karyocyte matures, acquiring azurophilic granules. Finally, platelets are produced by fragmentation of the megakaryocyte cytoplasm. Each megakaryocyte produces some 4000 platelets which are approximately 1–2 μm in diameter. Megakaryocytic maturation is divided into three stages: The megakaryoblast, promegakaryocyte and megakaryocyte.

DOI: 10.1201/9781003474432-4

Megakaryoblast

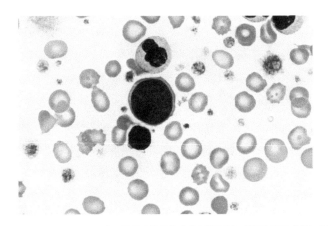

Megakaryoblast: Blood film from a patient with chronic myelogenous leukaemia, BCR-ABL1 positive, who has undergone splenectomy showing a circulating megakaryoblast in the peripheral blood (×1000).

The megakaryoblast is a large cell about 20–30 μm in diameter. It has a single oval or kidney-shaped nucleus, several nucleoli and basophilic non-granular cytoplasm.

Promegakaryocyte

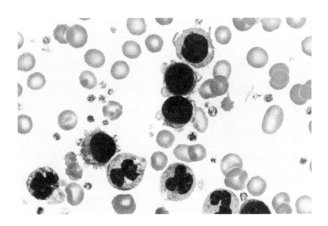

Promegakaryocytes: Peripheral blood film from the case above showing circulating promegakaryocytes. Note the cytoplasm budding (×1000).

The promegakaryocyte is larger than the megakaryoblast and has two to four nuclei with several nucleoli. The cytoplasm is basophilic and contains fine azurophilic granules.

Megakaryocyte

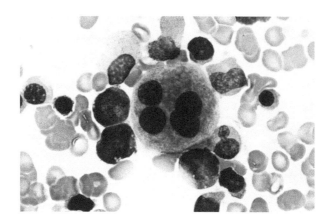

Megakaryocyte: Bone marrow showing a mature megakaryocyte (×1000).

The megakaryocyte is a large cell measuring 30–90 µm in diameter containing 8, 16 or 32 nuclei. The cytoplasm is less basophilic and shows diffuse azurophilic granulation.

Platelet abnormalities

Reactive thrombocytosis

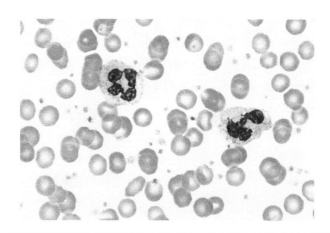

Reactive thrombocytosis: Peripheral blood film from an eight-month-child with juvenile rheumatoid arthritis with a platelet count of 1046 × 10⁹/L (×1000).

Large and giant platelets

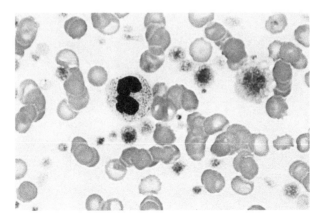

Large and giant platelets in a case of post splenectomy (×1000).

Seen in a case of post splenectomy (×1000).

Platelet aggregates

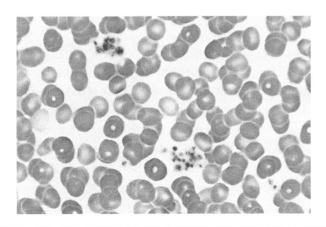

Platelet aggregates: Platelet aggregates in EDTA samples of peripheral blood usually result from difficulty in collection or less frequently from anti-platelet anti-EDTA antibodies. The presence of platelet aggregates result in an erroneously low platelet count (×1000).

Platelet aggregates in EDTA samples usually result from difficulty in collection or less frequently from anti-EDTA antibodies. The presence of platelet aggregates results in an erroneously low platelet count (×1000).

Platelet satellitism

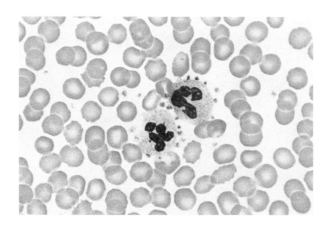

Platelet satellitism: This is a rarely seen phenomenon in which the platelets adhere to neutrophils. It occurs in EDTA blood resulting in an erroneously low platelet count. Its pathogenesis and significance are unknown (×1000).

A rarely seen phenomenon in which the platelets adhere to the neutrophils. It occurs in EDTA blood resulting in an erroneously low platelet count. Its pathogenesis and significance are unknown (×1000).

Thrombocytopenia

Thrombocytopenia is a frequent appearance amongst illborns, being found in 20–30% of all admissions to a neonatal intensive care ward. It is more common among infants with neonatal asphyxia, respiratory distress syndrome, pulmonary hypertension and meconium aspiration. The aetiology of the thrombocytopenia is not understood. The platelet life span is decreased while the megakaryocyte numbers are normal or increased. These features are also seen in infection, disseminated intravascular coagulation and immune/mechanical destruction.

Most infants with thrombocytopenia come to the attention of the neonatologist because of haemorrhagic symptoms: Petechiae, purpura, epistaxis or mucous membrane bleeding. Mechanisms of thrombocytopenia in neonates and children fall into two basic categories: Increased destruction and impaired or ineffective thrombopoiesis.

Thrombocytopenia due to increased destruction (ITP)

Thrombocytopenia due to increased destruction (ITP) is one of the most frequently seen examples of increased destruction. A typical history is bruising and petechiae appearing suddenly in a child who is in otherwise excellent health. The peak age for the diagnosis of ITP is 2–4 years. In childhood ITP, males and females are affected with equal frequency in contrast to adult ITP, in which females dominate by a 3:1 ratio. Often there is a history of a viral illness or vaccination one to three weeks prior to presentation.

The platelet count in these children is commonly <10 × 10⁹/L. The blood film should be carefully scanned for the presence of reactive lymphocytes as well as large platelets when a case of ITP is suspected.

In the majority of cases, ITP in children is an acute self-limiting disease resolving within six months whether or not therapy is given.

Thrombocytopenia due to impaired or ineffective thrombopoiesis

Thrombocytopenia secondary to a primary haematological process such as any of the following disorders: TAR syndrome, Fanconi anaemia, Bernard–Soulier syndrome, May–Hegglin anomaly, Wiskott–Aldrich syndrome. Thrombocytopenia can also be secondary to acquired disorders such as aplastic anaemia, bone marrow infiltration and drug or radiation-induced or secondary to platelet sequestration such as hypersplenism.

Amegakaryocytic thrombocytopenia (AMEGA)

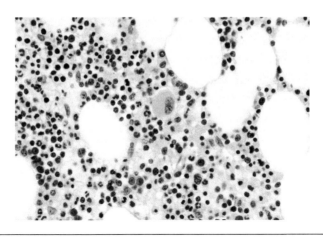

Amegakaryocytic thrombocytopenia: Bone marrow trephine showing a single hypolobulated megakaryocyte in the presence of normal granulopoiesis and erythropoiesis (H&E) (×1000).

Amegakaryocytic thrombocytopenia (AMEGA) occurs in infancy and early childhood. The mode of inheritance is either X-linked or autosomal recessive. AMEGA is a very rare disorder in which patients present with a petechial rash, bruising or bleeding in the first year of life. Mild to moderate anaemia and leucopenia may be present. Megakaryocytes in the bone marrow are either reduced in number or absent. Granulopoiesis and erythropoiesis are normal. The red cells may be macrocytic and the HbF increased. Between 20% and 40% of cases may develop aplastic anaemia in the first few years of life. Patients with AMEGA have a predisposition to develop acute leukaemia.

Bernard–Soulier syndrome (BSS)

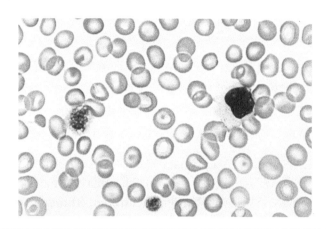

Bernard–Soulier syndrome: Peripheral blood film showing thrombocytopenia and giant platelets. Often the platelets are the size of small lymphocytes (×1000).

Bernard–Soulier syndrome (BSS) is inherited as an autosomal disorder. It is characterised by a moderate thrombocytopenia. The platelet counts range from 50–60 × 10^9/L, with giant forms present, many being the size of small lymphocytes. The platelets in BSS demonstrate both qualitative and quantitative defects in the glycoprotein 1b-V-1X complex within the platelet membrane. BSS platelets demonstrate normal aggregation in the presence of adenosine diphosphate (ADP), epinephrine (adrenaline), collagen and arachidonic acid, but do not aggregate in the presence of ristocetin.

Grey platelet syndrome (GPS)

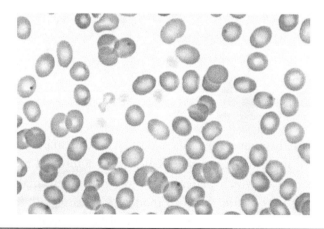

Grey platelet syndrome: Peripheral blood film showing large pale-staining and poorly granulated platelets (×1000).

Grey platelet syndrome (GPS) is inherited as an autosomal-dominant disorder. It is characterised by a moderate thrombocytopenia with large pale staining platelets on the Romanowsky-stained film. The platelets are deficient in α-granules. There is also a deficiency in storage proteins, platelet factor 4, thrombospondin, platelet-derived growth factor and β-thromboglobulin. These storage proteins may be increased in the serum, suggesting a defect in α-granule protein packaging within the megakaryocyte. The megakaryocytes are normal in number but poorly granulated. Patients with GPS have a prolonged skin bleeding time and hence a mild bleeding tendency.

May–Hegglin anomaly (MHA)

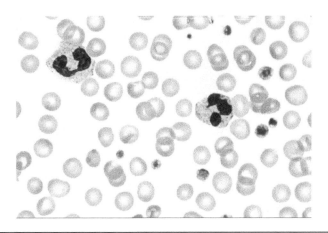

May–Hegglin anomaly: Peripheral blood film showing inclusions of RNA within the neutrophil cytoplasm as well as thrombocytopenia and large platelets (×1000).

May–Hegglin anomaly (MHA) anomaly is inherited as an autosomal-dominant disorder characterised by the presence of giant platelets, variable thrombocytopenia and RNA inclusion bodies within the cytoplasm of the neutrophils. Platelet function is also variable; it may be normal in some cases but impaired in others.

Thrombocytopenia with absent radii (TAR)

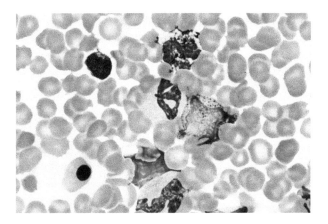

Thrombocytopenia with absent radii syndrome: Peripheral blood film from a newborn showing a leukaemoid reaction and thrombocytopenia (×1000).

Thrombocytopenia with absent radii (TAR) syndrome is inherited as an autosomal disorder. It is characterised by a thrombocytopenia and bilateral radial aplasia. The bone marrow shows decreased to absent numbers of megakaryocytes. Myelopoiesis and erythropoiesis are normal although a leucocytosis with counts of more than 100 × 10^9/L as well as the presence of immature myeloid forms may be present at birth. This leukaemoid reaction is transient and subsides spontaneously. Anaemia due to blood loss resulting from the thrombocytopenia may also be present.

Wiskott–Aldrich syndrome (WAS)

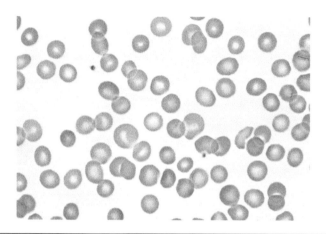

Wiscott–Aldrich syndrome: Peripheral blood film showing small platelets and thrombocytopenia (×1000).

Wiscott–Aldrich syndrome (WAS) is inherited as an X-linked disorder. It is characterised by thrombocytopenia with small platelets (note reduced MPV) that have a slightly reduced survival time. Thrombopoiesis is ineffective while megakaryocyte numbers range from normal to high. Immunodeficiency is also a feature of WAS. An inability to produce antibodies makes children with WAS susceptible to both bacterial and viral infections (e.g., herpes and warts). Eczema is also commonly seen. A positive DAT haemolytic anaemia may also occur in conjunction with WAS.

Thrombocytosis

The most frequently occurring causes of thrombocytosis in neonates and children are reactive. They include infection (bacterial and viral), surgery or trauma, haemorrhage, stress, inflammatory disease (rheumatoid arthritis), malignancies, chronic blood loss, the use of certain drugs and the use of cytokines. With any of the above, the degree of thrombocytosis usually parallels the degree of activity of the underlying condition.

Lymphoproliferative neoplasms

B lymphoblastic leukaemia/lymphoma

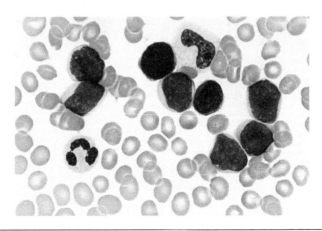

B-lymphoblastic leukaemia: Peripheral blood film showing blast cells with a high N/C ratio, fine to clumped chromatin pattern and inconspicuous nucleoli (×1000).

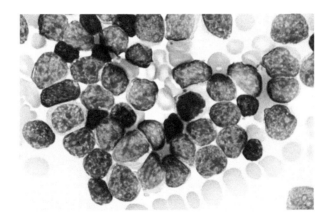

B-lymphoblastic leukaemia: Bone marrow showing a homogeneous infiltrate of lymphoblasts (×1000).

B-lymphoblastic leukaemia: Peripheral blood film showing blast cells with a high N/C ratio, fine to clumped chromatin pattern and inconspicuous nucleoli (×1000).

B-lymphoblastic leukaemia: Bone marrow showing a homogeneous infiltrate of lymphoblasts (×1000).

T-lymphoblastic leukaemia

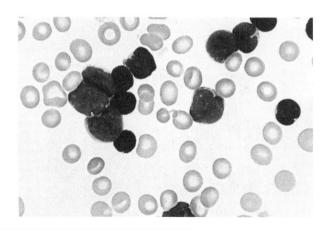

T-lymphoblastic leukaemia: Peripheral blood showing blast cells with a high N/C ratio, fine to clumped chromatin pattern, cleaved nuclei and inconspicuous nucleoli (×1000).

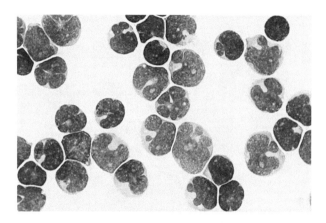

T-lymphoblastic leukaemia: Central nervous system relapse showing a heavy infiltrate of cleaved lymphoblasts (×1000).

Peripheral blood showing blast cells with a high N/C ratio, fine to clumped chromatin pattern, cleaved nuclei and inconspicuous nucleoli (×1000).

Central nervous system (CNS) relapse showing a heavy infiltrate of cleaved lymphoblasts (×1000).

A full account of lymphoproliferative neoplasms according to the WHO classification is beyond the scope of this paediatric text. However, when one is working in a large paediatric hospital, the majority of young children and even neonates who present with pancytopenia invariably is diagnosed with a lymphoproliferative neoplasm. The most common diagnosis is Precursor B lymphoblastic leukaemia.

Should the morphologist be reporting on the blood film from a young child with pancytopenia, always be mindful of the possibility that the child may have leukaemia. One must scan the blood film very carefully, scanning both the edges of the film looking for large cells which may be blast cells. Always be mindful of the fact that large cells will go to the edges of a manually spread blood film.

B lymphoblastic leukaemia/lymphoma is a disease of precursor B lymphoblasts. It occurs mainly in young children and approximately 75% of cases occurring in children less than six years of age while B lymphoblastic lymphoma has a median age of 20 years. The lymphoblasts range from those with a high N:C ratio, fine to clumped chromatin pattern with inconspicuous nucleoli and scanty basophilic cytoplasm to those that are heterogeneous in cell size and have a nuclear chromatin pattern varying from finely dispersed to coarsely condensed. Nuclear clefting, indentation and folding are characteristic and gross irregularities in shape are common. Nucleoli are nearly always present with variably in size and number. The amount of cytoplasm is variable and often abundant. The term 'B-lymphoblastic leukaemia' applies when there is involvement of the peripheral blood and bone marrow and the term 'B-lymphoblastic lymphoma' when there is significant nodal and extranodal involvement. The distinction between the two names is arbitrary.

Immunophenotype

Early-B ALL	TdT+, HLA-DR+, SIg−, cyt-μ−, CD10−, CD19+, CD22+, CD34+
Common B ALL	TdT+, HLA-DR+, SIg−, cyt-μ−, CD10+, CD19+, CD22−, CD34+
Pre-B ALL	TdT+, HLA-DR+, SIg−, cyt-μ+, CD10+, CD19+, CD22+, CD34−
B ALL	TdT−, HLA-DR+, SIg+, CD10−, CD19+, CD20+, CD22+, CD34−

T lymphoblastic leukaemia/lymphoma

T lymphoblastic leukaemia/lymphoma is a disease of precursor T lymphoblasts. T lymphoblastic leukaemia occurs more commonly in adolescents than in young children. It also occurs in adults of any age group. The lymphoblasts are small to medium in size with a high N:C ratio, moderately condensed chromatin pattern and inconspicuous nucleoli. The term 'T-lymphoblastic leukaemia' applies when there is involvement of the bone marrow and peripheral blood and the term 'T-lymphoblastic lymphoma' when there is significant nodal or extranodal involvement. The distinction between the two names is arbitrary.

Immunophenotype

TDT+, HLA-DR−, CD1a+, CD2+, CD3+, CD4+/−, CD5+, CD7+, CD8+/−

Index

*For Product Safety Concerns and Information please contact
our EU representative GPSR@taylorandfrancis.com Taylor & Francis
Verlag GmbH, Kaufingerstraße 24, 80331 München, Germany*

T - #0293 - 160425 - C114 - 254/178/6 - PB - 9781032753904 - Gloss Lamination